Swallow This

BY THE SAME AUTHOR

The Food Our Children Eat

Shopped

Bad Food Britain

What to Eat

Swallow This

Serving up the food industry's darkest secrets

JOANNA BLYTHMAN

FOURTH ESTATE • *London*

First published in Great Britain in 2015 by
Fourth Estate
An imprint of HarperCollins*Publishers*
1 London Bridge Street
London SE1 9GF

www.4thestate.co.uk

1 3 5 7 9 10 8 6 4 2

A catalogue record for this book is
available from the British Library

ISBN 978-0-00-754833-0

Printed and bound in Great Britain

In memory of Derek Cooper,
a fellow foot soldier in the food wars.

Contents

Introduction

Journalists don't like to be palmed off with half the story, but even though I had 25 years of food chain investigations under my belt, six books to my name, and a collection of awards and gongs on my trophy shelf, I had a sneaking suspicion that this was exactly what was happening. Unanswered, or only partially answered, questions about the food we consume each day nagged away at the back of my mind. How 'natural' is the process for making a 'natural' flavouring? What, exactly, is modified starch, and why is this ingredient in so many foods? What is done to pitta bread to make it stay 'fresh' for six months? Why, when I eat a supermarket salad, does the taste linger in my mouth for several hours after? Slowly but surely, I realised just how little information about food production methods is in the public realm, despite the best efforts of those of us who interrogate the inner workings of the industry.

Now this assessment might seem counterintuitive, after all, you would be right in thinking that food exposés are a staple ingredient in news headlines. The media attention lavished on food fraud in particular is not inconsiderable. Thanks to such revelations, we know, for example, that crooks have illegally fed a stream of horsemeat into some of our most popular processed meats. We suspect, with some justification, that such incidents are only the tip of an iceberg.

But my frustration, my sense of not quite getting to the bottom of the story, was more fundamental. Forget *illegal* activities in the food chain, what about the perfectly *legal* activities that go on every day behind the scenes? What do we know about them? I'm not talking about primary food producers, farmers and growers; what happens down on the farm and out in the fields. This link in our food chain is passably well policed and transparent. Nor am I talking about the abattoir where, once again, there are regular inspections, even the occasional undercover reporter from a vigilant animal welfare group, armed with a video camera. No, my growing preoccupation was just how pathetically little we really knew about processed food, the food that sits on supermarket shelves in boxes, cartons and bottles, everything that comes wrapped or packed in some way, food that has had something done to it to make it more convenient and ready-to-eat.

My interest was in not just the most clearly processed, most industrialised offerings, things like ready meals, chicken nuggets, oven chips and tinned soups, but also those that less obviously bear the stamp of the food factory: washed salads, smoothies, yogurt, cheese, cereal bars, butchered meat, fresh fish, bread, fruit juice, prepared vegetables, and so on. Many switched-on consumers try to avoid the former, but you would need to be a desert island hermit to steer clear of the latter.

Slowly but surely, factory-made food has come to occupy an ever more bloated position in our diet. You might find it all too easy to resist the lure of a turkey drummer, a ready meal, a lurid fruit 'drink', or a pappy loaf of standard white bread. You might even boycott the most obvious forms of nutritionally compromised, blatantly degraded offerings, and yet you will still find it hard to avoid the 6,000 food additives – flavourings, glazing agents, improvers, anti-caking agents, solvents, preservatives, colourings, acids, emulsifiers, releasing agents, antioxidants, thickeners, bleaching agents, sweeteners, chelators – and the undisclosed 'processing aids', that are routinely employed behind the scenes of contemporary food manufacture. That upmarket cured ham and salami, that 'artisan' sourdough loaf, that seemingly authentic Levantine halva, that 'traditional' extra mature, vintage Cheddar cheese, those supposedly health-promoting, rustic-looking breakfast cereals, those luxurious Belgian chocolates, those speciality coffees and miraculous probiotic drinks, those virginal yogurts that seem as pure as driven snow, those apparently inoffensive bottles of cooking oil, and much, much more may all have had a more intimate relationship with state-of-the-art food manufacture technology than we appreciate.

The curious thing about processed foods, be they of the crude type or the more sophisticated sort, is that their mode of production is an enigma. Of course, anything that comes in a box, tin, bag, carton or bottle has to bear a label listing its contents, and many of us have become experts at reading these labels to avoid ingredients with unnatural-sounding chemical connotations. But guess what? Many of the additives and ingredients that once jumped out at us from labels as flagging up something fake and unfathomable have quietly disappeared from listings.

Does this mean that their contents have improved? Possibly, but there is an alternative explanation. Over the last few years, many food companies have embarked on an operation dubbed 'clean label', with the goal of removing the most glaring industrial ingredients and additives from labels, replacing them with substitutes that sound altogether more benign. Many of the factory-made, processed foods on our shelves have discreetly undergone a before-and-after makeover, and many have also been relabelled with confidence-inducing buzzwords such as 'antioxidant', 'gluten-free', 'whole grain', 'more of', 'less' of, 'high in', 'low in', 'reduced sugar', etc., which psychologically prime us to infer that they bring an overall health benefit to our tables. It all comes together to make a seemingly informative chorus.

But when you try to dig deeper, as I wanted to do, to go beyond the label, you hit a wall of secrecy. How is a ready-to-eat cottage pie actually made? Why is there high fructose corn syrup in your steak and ale pie? How are zero-calorie sweeteners created? What makes those cherries in your fruit cake stay firm? Why are those peppers so shiny? Why would you need beef protein in a pork sausage? Expect to draw a blank.

Back in the days when food writers were stereotyped by processed food manufacturers and retailers as fluffy-headed scribes who could be enlisted to help sell their products, several big food companies opened their doors to them. They were given a selectively edited diplomatic tour of the processing facility, spending most of the visit well away from the din and distress of the factory floor in the relative calm of the development kitchen. Here they were expected to ooh and ah about the latest prepared dish soon to be shipped out to stores around the land, then write about it enthusiastically in magazines and supplements. Celebrity chefs 'consultants' were paid handsomely to lend their seal of approval to products churned out by industrial food companies, sprinkling on them the stardust that surrounds this much-admired profession.

This romancing of the food media stuttered to a halt when reservations about industrial food production practices reached critical mass and food scandals started to feature in news pages. In 1990, for instance, the Norfolk turkey king, Bernard Matthews, abruptly terminated a face-to-face interview with me in his office when I put to him questions about mechanically recovered meat, and asked to be shown round one of his windowless poultry sheds.

For at least the last decade, the big manufacturing companies that turn ingredients into products have kept a low profile. They take refuge in health and safety rules; factories are dangerous places after all. And they hide behind the creed of commercial confidentiality. We can't let our competitors know what's in our secret recipe, now can we? Fair enough, but also a perfect way to stonewall citizens who want to know just a little bit more about the genesis of their pulled pork pizza or their microwaveable veg pot.

Nowadays, manufacturers leave it to retailers to field any searching questions. Retailers in turn take shelter behind the will-sapping, call-centre pointlessness of the customer care line. Here the tactic is to drown callers in superfluous, mainly irrelevant material (long lists of allergens, calorie counts and so on) without answering any tricky questions. The most persistent enquirers may be treated to an edit-to-suit, off-the-peg customer reply letter from corporate HQ containing a bland, non-specific reassurance, such as: 'Every ingredient in this product conforms to quality assurance standards, EU regulations, additional protocols based on the tightest international requirements, and our own demanding specification standards ... blah de blah.' Basically, thank you and goodbye.

Few journalists nowadays bother approaching the press offices of our large food retailers and manufacturers unless they have a very specific, narrow query, such as 'Do you sell skipjack tuna caught in purse seine nets?' Any broader enquiry is likely to be met with a cloud of words more insubstantial than a breakfast waffle. Even then, they do not expect a prompt or particularly illuminating response. Relatively junior press office staff will log and note the query, and if it sounds potentially troublesome, pass it upstairs to their superiors. In this case, corporate affairs executives will be on the job, framing a carefully worded response, which, when you pare it down, discloses the barest possible substantive fact.

And if the truth were told, few people outside the world of food processing, journalists or otherwise, are in a position to pose pertinent questions anyway. You need to understand a bit about a subject in order to know what questions to ask, and the increasingly complex technologies used in contemporary food manufacturing are shrouded in mystery to all but industry initiates.

So I set out to put in the public domain more information about the mechanics of how factory food is made. Where to begin? By guaranteeing that the visits would be for background only, I managed to see inside some of the more open-minded manufacturing facilities, which was illuminating up to a point, except that these plants are so thoroughly industrial, that it was not easy to interpret what I was seeing, or work out which bits of the production process I wasn't being shown.

As far as general research went, using all the resources the internet has to offer, materially enlightening information was equally hard to come by. All the companies that supply ingredients to the food and drink manufacturing arena have a public or media website, accessible to anyone who bothers to look. These typically consist of a mixture of old press releases, business statistics – how many people we employ in how many countries, and so on – and Frequently Asked Questions. These public sites are conspicuously devoid of tangible facts. Their creators have clearly mastered the art of saying nothing much, at great length. All are designed to cast the company's activities in a flattering light.

Then there are separate sites, or subscriber-only areas of company sites, that share product knowledge and developments amongst industry insiders. These facilitate a deeper level of dialogue that is internal to the food manufacturing business; the trade talking to the trade. In particular, they allow the chemical industry to tell food manufacturers how our food can be shaped, engineered and redesigned. They offer practical case studies of how innovative modern ingredients, such as enzymes, nanoparticles, protein isolates, acidulants, permeates, cyclodextrins and sugar alcohols can revolutionise production, and offer technical 'solutions' to commonly encountered problems. Even then, when it comes to the nitty-gritty of what an ingredient, additive or process actually involves or does in a specific food or drink context, manufacturers are almost invariably urged to contact the company direct to discover what technical 'applications' the product in question might have for their business.

Such sites are very definitely do-not-disturb zones for industry outsiders. In fact, you need to pass through various hurdles to be allowed into the club. For instance, when I tried to subscribe to Innovadex, formerly known as Chemidex, the biggest online ingredient search engine for food and drink manufacturers, I received the following reply:

> Thank you for completing your registration with Innovadex. Access is not immediate and is dependent upon approval. Notification of your access will be sent within one business day. Innovadex.com is an internet-based resource designed specifically for use by chemists and formulators. Membership is restricted to validated institutional users of product information who are involved in the purchase and use of raw materials and ingredients.

Needless to say, my Innovadex subscription was not forthcoming, and it was the same story with the registered users-only sites of companies supplying our food manufacturers. Here you have to fill in a series of subscription application questions to establish your suitability. What is the name of your company? What is your company website? What sector are you in (meat, dairy, bakery, etc.)? Are you a manufacturer or retailer? What is your position and job title in the company (product developer, buyer, processor, etc.)? How many employees do you employ? What band does your annual turnover fall into? What school did you last attend? I'm joking about this last one, but unless you fit searching criteria, your subscription application goes no further.

What about dropping in on some of the global summits where food manufacturers network with 'visionary researchers', 'thought leaders' and 'horizon scanners' from leading ingredient suppliers? The same restrictions apply. You must be an approved industry insider of the vetted sort, and even if you are, the fee for attendance is pitched at a level (several hundreds, sometimes thousands of pounds) that only deep corporate pockets can contemplate. In food manufacturing, no one seems to blink at stumping up £1,999 for a conference pass, or paying £399 upwards for a workshop; and that's before VAT.

Just supposing you were enough of an anorak to want to read and digest meaty technical documents that would help cast light on what goes on behind the scenes of food manufacturing, you would have to pay handsomely for the privilege. For instance, a publication, such as 'Food Flavours & Flavour Enhancers: Market, Technical & Regulatory Insights', published by market researchers, Mintel, and Leatherhead Food Research, a leading food and drink industry research and development body, might fill us in on how these additives are used, and give us a steer on how much of them we all consume. But at £2,600 plus VAT, just like a Rolex, that's a rather exclusive purchase. In many different ways, food manufacturers and the global ingredients companies that supply them, operate a very effective apartheid system that bars anyone who doesn't belong. Glasnost is not a core operating principle of the factory food industry.

Fortunately for consumers, the food and drink industry is not a monolith, and not all companies believe that the public is best left in the dark. A couple of them very kindly provided me with a 'cover' that allowed me to pass through the security vetting and gain unprecedented access to material that has not previously been in the public realm. They helped me get closer to the beating heart of modern factory food production. This book is all about what I found there, and even to me, as a seasoned food journalist, it was an eye-opener.

In the first part, I have tried to set the scene of how the world of food and drink manufacturing operates, from the factory floor, to the supermarket sales floor, and at a cutting edge industry event. In the second part, I have laid out before you what, after all my research, I now consider to be the defining characteristics of this industry's products: food and drink that is sweet, oily, old, flavoured, coloured, watery, starchy, tricky and packed. Where possible, I have allowed the industry to speak for itself. Quotes are revealing. When a company offers manufacturers 'customised masking solutions for tastes you want to hide', or promises shelf life extension products that give foods a 'fresh-like' quality for several weeks, this gives you a clue to some of this industry's paramount concerns.

In as much as we are encouraged to think about the nitty-gritty of manufacturing, that is, not at all, we are led to believe that what goes on in food factories is essentially the same as home cooking, only scaled-up. Any such perception is self-serving, coy and to my mind, misleading. What you might see, after dipping into this book, is how radically different food manufacturing is in its concepts, goals, behaviours and ethos from any form of domestic food preparation. Unlike home cooks, food manufacturers are driven by innovation and novelty. They work not from a framework of time-honoured principles, but with a blank sheet. Each new product is, in industry-speak, a 'matrix', a never-ending jigsaw puzzle of possible elements, either chiselled out from natural ingredients, or entirely man-made, that can be arranged and rearranged, right down to the molecular level if necessary, then stuck together in various ways, and in numerous forms, to meet certain overriding goals. For product developers and food technologists, the professionals who design and create a never-ending stream of products, whole, raw, unprocessed foods present a shopping trolley of components to play around with.

So when the home cook decides to make a Bakewell tart, for instance, she or he looks out a recipe, puts together a line-up of well-established ingredients – raspberry jam, flour, butter, whole eggs, almonds, butter and sugar – and then bakes it in a tried-and-tested way. The factory food technologist, on the other hand, approaches this venerable confection from a totally different angle. What alternative ingredients can we use to create a Bakewell tart-*style* product, while replacing or reducing expensive ingredients – those costly nuts, butter and berries? How can we cut the amount of butter, yet boost that buttery flavour, while disguising the addition of cheaper fats with an inferior taste profile? What sweeteners can we add to lower the tart's blatant sugar content and justify a 'reduced calorie' label? How many times can we re-use the pastry left over from each production run in subsequent ones? What antioxidants could we throw into the mix to prolong the tart's shelf life? Which enzyme would keep the almond sponge layer moist for longer? Might we use a long-life raspberry purée and gel mixture instead of conventional jam? What about coating the almond sponge layer with an invisible edible film that would keep the almonds crunchy for weeks? Could we substitute some starch for a proportion of the flour to give a more voluminously risen result? Would powdered, rather than pasteurised liquid egg, stick less to the equipment on the production line? Could we use a modified protein to do away with the eggs altogether, or to mimic fat? And so on.

According to the Food and Drink Federation, a body that promotes the interests of companies active in the field, food and drink manufacturing is 'a great British success story'. Thanks to the steady stream of pre-prepared, convenience food it puts on our plates, the average proportion of household income spent on food has dropped from 50 per cent in 1914 to around 10 per cent in 2014. In fact, the UK now spends less on food than any country in the world, bar the USA.

We have been striding purposefully down this Anglo-American food path for decades. George Orwell clocked the trend back in 1937 in his book, *The Road to Wigan Pier*. 'The English palate, especially the working-class palate, now rejects good food almost automatically. The number of people who prefer tinned peas and tinned fish to real peas and real fish must be increasing every year', he wrote. He noted that in England at that time, a man over six feet was usually 'skin and bone and not much else', attributing this largely to 'the modern industrial technique which provides you with cheap substitutes for everything'. He warned in no uncertain terms where the move away from home-cooked, real food might lead us: 'We may find in the long run that tinned food is a deadlier weapon than the machine gun'.

How prescient Orwell was. Nowadays, the expression of our ongoing embrace of factory food in its myriad processed forms is rather different than in the 1930s, with an irony that would not be lost on him. A growing number of us are simultaneously overfed and undernourished, a crazy consequence of our reliance on food manufactured in an industrial setting. Whereas Orwell linked processed food consumption with excessive skinniness, today's six-foot-tall man, like most other citizens, will most likely be carrying a good few kilos of excess weight. These days, a disturbing 60 per cent of the UK population is overweight; a quarter of us are obese.

Are we leaping to an unjustified conclusion when we lay a significant part of the blame for obesity, chronic disease and the dramatic rise in reported food allergies, at the door of processed food? There are several a priori grounds for seriously examining this possibility. Firstly, food manufacturers combine ingredients that do not occur in natural food, notably the trilogy of sugar, processed fat and salt, in their most quickly digested, highly refined, nutrient-depleted forms. Might these modern constructions be addictive? That proposition is gaining airtime. Secondly, manufactured foods often contain chemicals with known toxic properties – although we are reassured that at low levels, this is not a cause for concern. Thirdly, the processed food industry has an ignoble history of actively defending its use of controversial ingredients, such as partially hydrogenated oils, long after well-documented, subsequently validated, suspicions have been aired.

The precautionary principle doesn't seem to figure prominently in the convenience food industry's calculations, and such is the lobbying power of this influential sector, it does not loom large in the deliberations of our would-be regulators either. If it did, then steering clear of manufactured products that are very likely to prejudice your health would be a lot easier. All through this book, you will read examples of potentially harmful ingredients and processes being used in food and drink manufacturing, yet statutory bodies fail to restrict them because they do not yet have full, incontestable certainty of damage.

I would like to be able to report that the powers-that-be are working away in the best interests of the population to curb the processed food industry's worst excesses. I would be delighted if the concerns I raise in this book could be swept away by strategic government action: better labelling, taxes on miscreant foods, and tighter industry surveillance. But I believe that hell will freeze over before the state takes radical action to protect us from the damage caused by processed food. Why? This industry is just so damn profitable.

The bottom line here is that there are already reasonable grounds to infer that a diet heavy in processed food is bad for us. We can wait for that contention to be 'proven', and the activities of the companies that sell unhealthy food to be restricted, or we can start operating our own personal precautionary principle by eating less of it, and cooking more of our own food from scratch.

This is not to say that there is no such thing as a healthy, wholesome manufactured food. I happily use many processed ingredients. Realistically, I am not likely to keep a house cow for milk, or make my own butter and cheese. Nor do I intend to grow my own grain and mill it into flour; although I know some inspiring people who do, and very much admire their commitment. I am a purchaser of bread, not a baker. I might, in a flush of enthusiasm for a new recipe, make some egg pasta from scratch, but usually, I'll buy it in a packet. I don't lie awake at night worrying about what effect canning might have on my anchovies or pilchards. I often grind my spices for a special dish because they are fresher and more aromatic that way, but pre-ground spices also sit usefully in my larder alongside other processed foods such as tomato paste, soy sauce, sesame oil, rosewater, olives, gherkins, oatcakes, mustard. When my mother no longer has any of her homemade marmalade or jam to give me, I'll gladly buy some. My salads contain seeds that have been sprouted by someone other than me. Although I am intellectually enthused by the fashion for fermentation, I remain a more likely candidate for buying sauerkraut than making it. While I fully appreciate that it is possible to cure your own bacon, I'm just too lazy to try it.

In short, I have absolutely no intention of becoming a food neurotic, or living in splendid isolation as a Trappist monk. Like most of us, I am not always in control of what I eat, so I have to settle for the best option in the circumstances. Sometimes, I might be organised enough to bring my own food on a long journey, knowing that in quality terms, it will be streets ahead of anything I can buy, not to mention cheaper. But other times I still have to pick up lunch from a takeaway, trust my local delicatessen to make a reasonable quiche or sandwich, or politely eat a meal that I would never choose. I am also a restaurant critic, reviewing everything from chains to fine dining establishments on a weekly basis. Doing this job would be impossible if I was a purist, someone who took the attitude that my body is a temple that can never be sullied by processed food in any shape or form. I do not beat myself up if I can't meet my highest aspirations for eating good food on a daily basis. I am a pragmatist. Food is my love, not my enemy. I will not allow my professional knowledge of how it is produced to spoil my appetite for it.

Yet what I choose to eat and drink starts from the overarching principle that natural ingredients in their least processed forms have an inbuilt, effortless integrity that make them the best basis for a body and soul-sustaining life. Natural foods are brilliantly conceived and intricate little packages wherein every nutrient works in a companionable 'one for all, and all for one' synergy. When we prepare and eat natural foods, their wise completeness translates into palpable health benefits. Nutritionally speaking, the whole apple does much more for us than the apple juice, or the apple crumble, or the apple and oat breakfast bar, or the apple-flavoured gum, and it's hard to overeat whole apples. Manufactured foods, by contrast, are put together by people who, although indisputably smart and capable, do not have Nature's all-embracing, all-seeing intelligence. This is why so many of the products manufacturers create share the capacity to shorten our lifespans.

I honestly didn't set out to put you off eating anything that comes in a bottle, jar, packet, tin, tube, carton or polystyrene container, but when you read about certain practices and procedures used to make some of our most popular foods, this might somewhat dull your appetite for a few products. My message is not the comfortable one that the UK Department of Health wants to convey with its 'eatwell plate', which conspicuously promotes many popular processed foods and drinks – sweets, biscuits, cake, cornflakes, baked beans, flavoured yoghurts, sliced white bread, even a can of cola, and crisps – as part of a 'balanced diet'. Nor are the sentiments that run through this book in tune with the 'Don't Cook, Just Eat!' campaign so loudly promoted by purveyors of fast food, with eye-grabbing posters in the windows of takeaways up and down the land. Their self-styled 'anti-cooking manifesto' urges us to 'liberate' ourselves from its 'tyranny' by letting 'professionals do the work'.

Leave food to the professionals? Once you have digested the information in the pages that follow, you may understand why I am unable to oblige. Somehow, I feel more affinity with the message of the mysterious graffiti artist in Cologne who superimposes his or her own home cooking recipes on fast-food billboards, so that instead of seeing a Big Mac advert, for example, passers-by will spot the ingredients needed to make spaghetti with meat sauce, or a courgette rice casserole. These days, cooking is a powerful political statement, a small daily act of resistance that gives us significantly more control of our lives.

PART ONE

How the processed food system works

1

Why it all tastes the same

I am not a fan of convenience food, a sentiment rooted in a formative early experience. As a small child in the 1960s, I was captivated by the TV advert for one of the first generation of ready meals: the Vesta chicken curry. I seem to remember that it had beautiful sari-clad dancing girls, and all the thousand-and-one-nights exoticism so sumptuously on show in Alexander Korda's spectacular film, *The Thief of Bagdad*. Revisiting the Vesta advert now, with a more cynical adult eye, it would doubtless look laughably lame, but at the time, it had me spellbound.

In my home we ate almost no convenience food. Either my mother or grandmother cooked, more or less from scratch; this was the way most people ate until the 1970s. So I waged a long, attritional campaign to buy Vesta chicken curry, exercising what food advertisers now call 'pester power'. Neither the adults in the household, nor my older, wiser sister, shared my enthusiasm. I pleaded persistently with my mother who repeatedly blocked my requests. 'If you got it, you wouldn't like it really' she tried to convince me, to no avail. Then one night – bingo! – my parents were going out, and by way of compensation and a Saturday night treat, I was allowed to choose my own meal. My mother was worn down, and caved in. At last, I would get to taste the much longed-for Vesta curry! What's more, I'd even get to eat it on my lap while watching telly! In a household where we all sat down together for breakfast and evening meal, with the TV switched off, this departure from custom felt thrillingly subversive.

I'll never forget the crushing disillusionment I felt at the gulf between the TV advert, the imagery on the packaging, and the reality. The box showed an almond-eyed, bejewelled beauty bearing a generous plateful of something that looked enticingly glossy and brown, set on a bed of pearly white rice. But what I had on my lap was about half as much in quantity as I had expected, and the curry bit looked pretty much like dog food, or worse, something you'd been taught to step around if you saw it lying on the pavement.

I had to tough it out though. Maybe it would taste better than it looked; I didn't want to give anyone the opportunity to say 'We told you so'. But after a couple of mouthfuls, I was defeated, and had to admit that I just couldn't eat it. Fortunately, my grandmother was hovering around, with the comforting Plan B of cheese on toast already in mind.

I should point out that I was, perhaps, a rather unusual six-year-old: I had eaten curry and enjoyed spicy food. A family friend had once been in Pakistan and he had learned to make 'Indian' food that actually tasted like something you'd eat on the subcontinent, or so he said. In retrospect, since this was decades before the painstaking Madhur Jaffrey and Rick Stein age of grinding your own spices, I imagine he used the then ubiquitous ready-made Vencat curry powder, but what he cooked for us did, nevertheless, give us a hint of what home-cooked Indian food might taste like, enough for me to see instantly that Vesta curry, with its brown Windsor soup-like gloop, was something else entirely.

To backtrack here, Vesta, the pioneering ready meal brand, was already pushing a sales pitch that was to become all too familiar to British consumers. Its 'lavish' chicken curry came 'complete with an authentic curry sauce'. It was 'ready prepared by Vesta for you to cook' by 'expert chefs who have done the hard work for you'. OK, it was a slowcoach of a product by today's ping-of-a-microwave standards, taking 20 minutes to reheat, but that seductive labour-saving promise, combined with prominent claims of authenticity and the skill of a professional chef, is still the central plank in processed food marketing today. The ready meals entrepreneur, Sir Gulam Noon, summed up the industry's vision of itself when he told the *Financial Times* that he 'changed the palate of the nation, and broke the housewife's shackles from the kitchen'.

These days, convenience foods have certainly moved on from the Vesta days, both in terms of their technical sophistication and the claims advanced for their 'realness'. In the ready meal category, lasagne and chicken tikka are now the two best sellers. But I have yet to encounter a ready meal that tastes a lot, or even a little, like homemade food. They have improved from the Vesta days, but freed from their packaging and reheated, they generally remind me of the dispiriting hot meals dished up by budget airlines. That sticky brownness, that larger-than-life tinned tomato soup aroma, those uniform textures and consistencies, those starch-stiff ecru sauces, the predictable high tone twinning of sweet with salty, and the consequent thirst that surely follows; for me, ready meals are a sorry apology for real food.

I am forced to revisit this prejudice at regular intervals, however, when newspapers ask me to investigate a particular convenience food category – value, low-calorie, children's, free-from, for instance – and the claims made on their packaging. And trust me, there are legions of products to investigate. Looking at the chilled category alone, by 2013, UK-based food companies were manufacturing over 12,000 different chilled food recipes. This is a big business – over £10 billion a year – which represents some 13% of the UK's total retail food market. Within this grand total, ready meals are by far the largest sales category. The UK ate its way through 3 billion of them in 2012.

The only way to investigate ready meals properly is to buy a batch of comparable products from a variety of different retailers, and take them home to study in depth; it's not something that you can do easily in the supermarket aisle. The ingredients listing is obviously the first port of call, and these days, because processed foods such as ready meals are often complex, multi-ingredient products, these lists can run to several paragraphs of tiny print that's more or less impossible to read without some sort of magnification; unless, that is, you happen to have 20/20 vision.

Editors often want a description of how each product looks and tastes, so I remove them from their packaging and reheat them in the oven or pot. Now, perhaps if you eat them regularly, the sight and smell of warm, bubbling convenience meals will set your gastric juices flowing, but for people like me who aren't, they are strikingly different from the home-prepared equivalent. For starters, they often have a quite powerful odour, one that tends to hang around in the bin, sink and dishwasher long after the contents are gone.

Of course all food, including home-prepared food, makes itself known to the nasal passages to a greater or lesser extent, but usually in a pleasant, appealing way. Yet when you compare a selection of processed foods, you start noticing that they have particularly distinctive smells, or rather, a curiously similar portfolio of smells.

Now, according to Greencore, one of the largest chilled food manufacturers, the UK chilled food industry is 'the most advanced in the world because of its high standards, rigorous safety and management systems and the sheer quantity of exciting new recipes which it develops constantly'. That would make you think that there is a rich diversity amongst all the convenience foods on our shelves. But when I opened them in my kitchen, I found that I could easily classify my ready meals into odiferous families, a bit like houses of cards: aces, spades and so on. First there's the 'red' family, that's the hot tomato/pizza/lasagne/tomato and basil soup/'med' veg bunch. Next up, there's the 'brown' family, think of cottage pie/steak and kidney/casserole/stew/Peking duck, chow mein noodles and everything sold with a barbecue label. In the 'beige' family, variously labelled breadcrumbed/battered products share a strong resemblance, a particularly haunting, almost acrid oily aroma that soon impregnates the oven and lingers thereafter, irrespective of whether they are fish, meat or vegetable-based. The all-out attention-grabbers are the Indian-themed dishes, whose spices give them just enough personality to distinguish them from the others, although they otherwise share many similar characteristics.

When it comes to tasting ready meals, the flavour profiles are every bit as monotone as the smells. Tasted blind and mashed up to disguise any tell-tale texture, one might easily mix up a sausage casserole with barbecue spare ribs, or confuse Mexican chicken fajitas with sweet and sour chicken. Why is this?

It all began to fall into place when I was in the test kitchen of a ready meals factory, where food technologists check the taste and 'visuals' (appearance) of the day's output to ensure that they conform to a tight specification. 'The objective', one executive explained. 'is to see that the consumer gets the same taste experience every time'. Now this explained a lot. When you stop to think about it, home-cooked food varies all the time. For a kick-off, it reflects the cook's mood. Anyone who cooks can testify to how an oft-made recipe can turn out differently, depending on your mental state; harassed and rushed perhaps, serene and calm maybe, or even distracted and not fully engaged. Patiently caramelised onions one day can be burnt threads the next. There's a fine line between a custard sauce that obligingly coats the back of the spoon, and a bowlful of curdled egg.

The ingredients for home cooking also vary in subtle but palpable ways. One brand of tinned tomatoes doesn't give quite the same result as another. Lemons yield variable amounts of juice. Some bunches of herbs can be more aromatic than others, some spices fresher. Seasons make their presence felt too. Fresh summer garlic is sweet and subtle; the same bulb, stale, overwintered and used in March, can have a blunderbuss effect on a dish. Stewing beef bought from the supermarket, and encased in plastic with gases to keep it looking ruby red, will cook differently from the same cut, simply wrapped in waxed and brown paper, purchased from an independent butcher.

You may be a huge fan of your mum's homemade steak pie but have to admit that, this week, it didn't taste quite as great as usual. Or the opposite might be the case. One night, for no apparent reason, a familiar stir-fry suddenly seems to have acquired a mystery X factor. Was it that the peppers were less watery? Was the oil hotter because of that phone call? Was it down to the noticeable freshness and lack of fibre in that particularly good-looking root ginger?

It's the intrinsic variation that makes home-cooked food eternally interesting, but variation is the sworn enemy in industrial food processing. Indeed, all the systems put in place by manufacturers of ready meals and other convenience food lines are geared to eliminating it. The whole purpose of the endeavour is to iron out every possible high and low, and produce a totally standard product that always looks and tastes identical, 365 days of the year. As one government food safety manual puts it: 'To achieve a consistent product with the same appearance, flavour, shelf life, etc., it is important that the ingredient quantities, quality and the processing steps are always the same'.

The lengthy process of achieving this begins with the food manufacturer's shopping list. The aim here is to have maximum control over ingredients, to ensure that they are always identical. On an industrial scale, this means buying in ingredients to a very tight specification from specialised companies. Surprising though it might sound to the home cook for whom ingredient preparation is probably the largest component of the cooking effort, food manufacturers carry out little or no preparation of raw ingredients. Instead they buy them in substantially pre-prepared. So, contrary to the notion that ready meals and other convenience foods are brought to you by a company that does all the hard work, it would be more accurate to say that they come from a company that 'cooks' products made with a list (often long) of ingredients and sundry additives that have already undergone some form of preparation by several other companies. In other words, the company that appears to be saving you work (usually a supermarket), is devolving that work to another company (a food manufacturer), which in turn gets other companies (food processors) to do the prep for it. These processors, in turn, may be quite remote from the primary food producers: farmers and growers.

The convenience food chain that supplies the consumer is made up of many links, links that often cross continents. In food manufacturing logic, this elongated chain is not at all crazy, quite the opposite. After all, the basis of any automated industrial manufacturing, be it cars or chicken tikka, is breaking down all the necessary production stages into component parts that can be carried out by separate teams on the assembly line.

The Chilled Food Association presents its industry's products as 'local' because 'virtually all chilled prepared foods are made in the UK', but the ingredients used to make the finished products are often anything but. It quotes one development chef as saying: 'Food should be simple, well cooked and flavoursome, with minimal amount of handling. It is also essential to use the best available ingredients to hand and promote local produce wherever possible.' A statement somewhat at odds with industry recruitment literature, which describes 'sourcing fresh ingredients globally from carefully chosen suppliers' as a key part of the job.

In fact, the food manufacturer's shopping list is thoroughly international. When an ITV *Tonight* investigation, Food

Facts and Fiction, commissioned a UK food technologist with extensive experience of food manufacturing to make a very traditional British-sounding lamb hotpot ready meal of the type commonly sold by supermarkets, he came up with a product made from 16 ingredients, sourced from ten different countries, including New Zealand lamb, Israeli carrots, Argentinian beef bones and Majorcan potatoes.

Irrespective of which country they are buying from, if food manufacturers can buy an ingredient in frozen form, they will. That may seem surprising, even counterintuitive, given that they often go on to sell them chilled as 'fresh', but freezing is seen by food processors, quite correctly, as the safest way of storing ingredients to protect them against any food poisoning risk. Frozen ingredients are also easy for industrial food manufacturers to handle. They don't arrive at the delivery bay with a stopwatch ticking, needing to be cooked promptly. Instead they can be, and are, stored for months, even years, and brought out as and when they are needed. So most of the meat, fish and vegetables arrive at the factory gate in a frozen state, already months, possibly years, old.

By buying in frozen food, manufacturers liberate their purchasing from the vagaries of the seasons and price fluctuations, and benefit from buying ingredients in frozen bulk on a global market. So, unless the label specifies otherwise, it's highly probable, for instance, that the chicken in your ready meal was purchased frozen from either Thailand or Brazil. Around 40 per cent of the chicken we eat in the UK is imported, almost all of it destined for food processing or catering. If required, large chicken exporters in these countries will also obligingly supply that frozen chicken pre-cooked, and/or 'marinated': injected with water, cornflour, salt, and even other flavourings. Few consumers notice the tell-tale label description ('cooked marinated chicken breast') not unreasonably assuming that when a product contains chicken, that means 100 per cent chicken, probably British, the sort you'd cook at home, with nothing else added.

It's an eye-opener to see the ingredient storage zones of food factories. In a typical operation, almost all the meat, be it chicken, lamb, pork or beef, is bought in frozen. So before it can be used it has to be defrosted for five to six minutes. Don't for a second imagine that in big food manufacturing plants there are lines of people patiently peeling mounds of carrots and potatoes. In your typical industrial-scale factory, 80–90 per cent of all fresh vegetables are purchased in frozen form.

As anyone who cooks from scratch knows, many savoury recipes begin with chopping onions and finely mincing garlic, but food manufacturers do away with all that fuss. Instead they typically use pre-peeled frozen onions. These are purchased, usually from Poland (which seems to have captured the EU market in onion peeling) and despatched to another factory to be defrosted, chopped into 10 millimetre dice, or sliced, frozen once more, then re-supplied ready for use, wrapped in a plastic sleeve inside cardboard boxes. You'll never see a bulb or clove of garlic in a food manufacturing factory either, as it is commonly sourced (sometimes from Europe, usually from China) pre-chopped and frozen, or in a processed purée form.

Potatoes – now there's another labour-intensive vegetable – similarly arrive at the factory frozen and pre-sliced to a specified thickness, or cut into neat 20 millimetre cubes.

While chefs and home cooks routinely stump up for fresh leafy herbs, appreciating the fragrance and vitality they bring to a dish, food manufacturers like a shortcut. A stroll through the food manufacturer's 'fridge' will show you boxes of frozen ones, pre-chopped by some other food processor in a distant factory. And guess what, they are nothing like the fresh equivalent. So why use them? 'Frozen herbs have a better kick, or flavour profile', one manufacturing executive told me, but no self-respecting chef or home cook would put up with the ready-to-use herbs (from Germany) that I saw. They looked grey-green and even the coriander had none of the fragrance that this herb so reliably brings to a dish; in fact, it smelt of nothing. But food manufacturers like prepped ingredients like these because, from their point of view, buying in prepared ingredients is actually ultra-responsible because they come from factories specially geared up to handle them, where the skills needed, and the risks posed, are quite different from those in their own process.

Food manufacturers apply the same logic to cooking fruits and vegetables. Why would they bother with time-consuming, laborious preparation, after all, when they can buy them in frozen and ready to use? They only need to place an order, and pallet-loads of pre-fried or grilled aubergines, peppers and courgettes, sliced to the ideal dimensions for your roasted Mediterranean vegetable pizza, will be delivered to the loading bay. Why would they muck around setting up a factory line for the scratch preparation of fresh aromatics for your Thai curry when they can source ginger already sliced into julienne strips, lime leaves already 'milled' into specks, and 'nuggets' of pulped chilli – all frozen? In food manufacturing terms, it is economic lunacy to pay someone in the UK to remove the zest from real fruits for a cheesecake, when you can buy in frozen lemon, orange and lime zest that has been mechanically removed, in a dedicated citrus processing plant, in another country. But this remorseless logic also helps explain why the resulting pizza, curry and cheesecake retain only a faint, blurry memory of the freshly prepared equivalent. These pre-processed labour-saving ingredients are simply not fresh, and storage has robbed them of their initial sparkle.

In the food manufacturer's ingredient store, you get a further insight into why processed convenience foods don't taste convincingly like their home-cooked equivalent. In the same way that you will never see a stray onion skin lying around a ready meals factory, you're extremely unlikely to see an eggshell either. Eggs are supplied to food manufacturers in many forms, but almost never in their original packaging. Instead, they come in powders, with added sugar, for instance, or as albumen-only special 'high gel' products for whipping. Liquid eggs will be pasteurised, yolk only, whites only, frozen or chilled, or with 'extended shelf life' (one month), whatever is easiest. They may be liquid, concentrated, dried, crystallised, frozen, quick frozen or coagulated. Manufacturers can also buy in handy pre-cooked, ready-shelled eggs for manufacturing products like Scotch eggs and egg mayonnaise, or eggs pre-formed into 300-gram cylinders or tubes, so that each egg slice is identical and there are no rounded ends. These hardboiled, tubular eggs are snapped up by companies that make sandwiches. Manufacturers can also take their pick from bespoke egg mixes, ready to use in everything from quiches and croissants to glossy golden pastry glazes and voluminous meringues. And there is always the cheaper option of using 'egg replacers' made from fractionated whey proteins (from milk). No hurry to use them up either; they have a shelf-life of 18 months.

Some ingredients used by food manufacturers are recognisable to home cooks: products such as aseptic tomato paste, a cooked tomato liquid, aren't so different from cartons of passata you might keep at home, for example. True, they come in shuddering foil packs with the dimensions of a clothes dryer in a launderette, yet the contents aren't dissimilar. But alongside these scaled-up items is a collection of ingredients that you won't find in any domestic larder. Instead, you'll find products designed for particular factory purposes. If, for instance, you needed to make a batter at home, you would most likely start with flour and eggs, but manufacturers turn to ready-to-mix batters, or 'reliable coating systems' as they are known in the trade, specially formulated to produce identikit results in factory-scale production; everything from 'pre-dusts' and 'adhesion batters' to fritter mixes with a 'cake-like interface' and 'ovenable systems' designed for reheating in the microwave.

Why not just mix a fresh batter from scratch? As one supplier of batters explains:

> Meats, poultry, vegetables and other organic substrates can vary widely in moisture level, fat and protein content. The degree of denaturisation, surface irregularities and variations in the expansion and type of protein may also come into play. The appropriate batters can help offset the effects of processing variables such as line speed, age and brand of processing machinery, water quality, set-up time, the method of reconstitution used and the amount of breading pick-up.

Strip away the characteristically industrial language of food manufacturing here, and what this means is that whether you are talking about the batter on your haddock goujons, chicken dippers or onion rings, a pre-mix guarantees uniform results, day in, day out.

Where a home cook would use breadcrumbs, manufacturers use lots of specially devised breadcrumb-like products, a necessary component of many ready meals and other convenience foods, everything from the crunchy topping on your cauliflower cheese meal-for-one through fish fingers to chicken Kievs. Indeed, they have their pick of a whole range of breadcrumb-like coatings that come in a variety of hues (due to natural or artificial colours), with different textures (from light and crispy to hard and crunchy), and in different crumb sizes. No need ever to bother with a loaf of bread.

Rather than making potato gnocchi from freshly boiled potatoes, flour and egg, the way your Italian nonna used to do (what a hassle!), food manufacturers can just add an egg and water solution to a tub of pre-seasoned, roller-dried potato flakes, designed especially for this purpose, in a mix that already contains added emulsifiers, stabilisers, citric acid, antioxidants – all to oil the wheels of the industrial process – and carrot extract, the latter to give the beige-grey dough a more wholesome colour.

Of course, any well-stocked home cook's kitchen has a store cupboard of ingredients that add additional flavour dimensions to food. Salt and pepper, naturally, and then things like soy sauce, spices, sesame oil, mustard and vinegar, but manufacturers can call on a number of shortcut ingredients, available only to the trade, to do the job. You will see the odd tub of ground spices in the ready meals factory, but in food processing, few ingredients are that simple. Instead there are glazes, seasoning mixes, coaters, rubs and marinades. To an optimist, these might sound quite normal, but they are far from it. They are what's called in the business 'flavour technology systems' or 'flavour delivery systems': products specially formulated to encapsulate the aroma and taste of natural food in a handy, ready-to-use form, either dry, or in liquid form as part of a 'liquid flavour system'.

From a food manufacturer's perspective, why mix together several different seasonings, aromatics and condiments when you can buy one customised product that will give your basic ingredients exactly the twist you want? Barbecue glazes, for instance, come Cajun, honey roast, smoky, hot and spicy, or Deep South-style. Pre-cooked, water-injected, defrosted chicken can be 'marinated' or 'rubbed' with a whole list of them – Chinese, Moroccan, Tandoori, Thai, Mexican, Italian, Creole and more – to imbue the same bland meat with a veritable United Nations of food manufacturing personality.

While a home cook would need to marinate meat for several hours, or even overnight, with an off-the-peg marinade, manufacturers can achieve that just marinated look in minutes.

Forget the faff of grinding spices, or pulverising aromatics. Food manufacturers prefer to buy in ready-made 'cuisine pastes' from companies who understand 'the total requirements of manufacturers of savoury foods, providing complete, tailored solutions for a wide range of applications'. As the marketing blurb for one such company expresses it, 'our chef quality range of savoury ingredients deliver premium taste profiles and are dry blended to make your production process easier'.

A tub of ready-made pepper coating can be used to create an attractive crust, like that on a well-seasoned steak, or jerked chicken, as a flavouring for couscous and pasta salad, or to smarten up a flabby, defrosted salmon steak. Pass pallid poultry pieces through a machine that sprays on caramel before you cook it, and it will take on the Miami beach lifeguard bronze of a home-roast joint. A touch of liquid ham and cheese flavouring, incorporated into other liquid ingredients, will make your spaghetti carbonara smell particularly savoury. A hint of fish flavouring will reintroduce the memory of taste into the anodyne prawn in the middle of your sushi roll.

The composition of the products manufacturers use to flavour and lend personality to ready meals and other convenience foods varies but, in a nutshell, they bear only the most distant notional similarity to those traditionally available to the home cook, not least because they are often multi-ingredient items in their own right. Whatever their name and supposed ethnic identity, the master key recipe for these prêt-à-porter flavouring shortcuts doesn't vary that much either. Whether wet or dry, it is hard to escape the same old roll call of starches, gums, sweeteners and salt, along with synthesised flavourings and colourings. In one typical supermarket Chinese-style pork rib ready meal, the glaze alone contains 17 ingredients: sugar, salt, cornflour, dried glucose syrup, tomato, garlic and beetroot powders, spices, guar gum, vegetable oil, and more.

But to food manufacturers, this custom-made shopping list makes total business sense. Why, for instance, would you shell out for butter when you can instead dose your recipe with 0.02 per cent butter extract that will, as one flavour company promises, give your products a 'characteristic butter flavour ... [that] works well with bakeries, confectionery, candies, ice cream, popcorn, cereals, dressings [and] combines well with vanilla and cocoa flavour'? Or, there is always the option of using butter powder. Described by one company that makes it as 'a powdery, homogeneous and free-flowing cream to yellow powder', it is manufactured by spray-drying a mixture of butter, maltodextrins (starch) and milk proteins; a real boon to manufacturers who want an up-market 'made with butter' promise on their product label, but who don't want to fork out for the real thing. Butter is an expensive ingredient as far as food manufacturers are concerned. When you are churning out hundreds of tonnes of product a day, even a small reduction in the quantity you use can reduce ingredient costs significantly.

And why clog up your cold storage area with vats of real cream when you can use a 'powdery, homogeneous and free flowing cream to yellow powder with a cream taste and smell' that doesn't need to be chilled, and takes up a fraction of the factory space?

To a manufacturer whose constant concern is reducing or at least containing costs in the face of regular price rises in raw materials, it seems quite logical to use, say, a powder made from freeze-dried apricots, blended with some type of starch, that smells just enough like the fresh fruit to pass muster in your Danish pastries or yogurt, rather than much more expensive fresh apricots, or frozen apricot pulp.

From water-injected poultry and powdered coagulated egg, to ultra-adhesive batters and pre-mixed marinades, the raw materials in industrial food manufacturing are rarely as simple as most of us would like to think. In fact, they commonly share quite complicated back-stories of processing and intervention that their labels don't reveal. Indeed, they are predicated on ingredients that are processed, comprised versions of the real thing, far removed from their original forms.

The undisclosed hidden history of their ingredients helps explain why ready meals manufactured in factories cannot hold a candle to the competently homemade equivalent, prepared in a domestic or restaurant kitchen. It also sheds light on why supposedly different ready meals from different retailers taste so similar. The big supermarket chains that sell us these products share the same manufacturers. These manufacturers, in turn, share the same pool of ingredient suppliers. The specifications our multiple retailers give to manufacturers may vary marginally – one might prefer a runnier stew, the other a stickier one – but the industrial systems they are locked into leave little leeway for genuine variety. One conveyor belt, on a given day of the week, is dedicated to meals for Asda or Tesco, while another does pretty much the same thing for M&S and Sainsbury's. One chain might specify a certain ingredient, say free-range pasteurised egg rather than the caged-hen equivalent, but no manufacturer can afford to alter their production system on request, especially when they very rarely have the security of proper contracts from retailers, only short-term agreements. So like a subscription to over-hyped satellite TV channels, the selection of ready meals on supermarket shelves, despite the apparent diversity, is surprisingly homogenous in terms of its contents.

And if the larder used by manufacturers is, shall we say, samey, what of the production method? In the context of food processing, the word cooking merits permanent parenthesis because the techniques used are so radically different from the time-honoured equivalent as understood by cooks down the ages. Any good domestic cook making the meat ragù for a pasta dish, for instance, would begin by browning onions and mince before adding the liquid ingredients, in order to deepen the flavour. In food mass production, you can forget pre-browning. All the ingredients will be measured into one gigantic, temperature-controlled industrial vat and bubbled up for a specified time until they form a stew-like mass. Add a dash of extract of this, and powder of that, and hey presto, you have the recipe for a meat layer. A dose of caramel will compensate for the missing taste, colour and aroma that natural browning would have given the dish. A little added thickener, in one form or another, usually from cheap sweet starches and sticky gums, will give the illusion of the natural viscosity found in the patiently made traditional article. All that remains is to have the mixture spewed into plastic cartons, along with the other manufactured white sauce and pasta components, and passed through blisteringly hot, cavernous steam-injected ovens to ensure that your lasagne or pasta bake remains soft for reheating. A rapid cooling in a spiral chiller, a mechanical conveyor system that moves food through a continuous chilling process, and the job is done.

What you have here is a streamlined production system of assembly, amalgamation, fusion, combination and transformation by heat that very efficiently flattens out any slight lingering personality in already anonymous, much compromised ingredients. No wonder ready meals taste so spookily similar. If the beauty industry is in the business of selling hope in a jar, the factory food industry is in the business of selling hope in a plastic carton, under a cardboard sleeve. It promises us something near-instant and edible that tastes more or less like real, home-cooked food – a promise that it is structurally unable to deliver.

2

On the factory floor

I now realise that I was naïve, but there was a time when I expected food processing companies to joyously announce their existence. I suppose that I had imagined factories with household names above the door, and proud signage explaining what they do. 'Smith & Sons: delicious meals in minutes', that sort of thing. I can't think why I clung to this idea, because come to think of it, I had never stumbled upon any that fitted that bill.

It was only when I started searching out the companies that process our food that I understood why: they prefer to keep a low profile, on industrial estates in amongst other anonymous, big box industrial units. Such locations give them the space and freedom to operate day and night. There are no immediate neighbours to complain about noise or smells. Heavy lorries can come and go, without drawing the ire of the local community.

Considering the volume of products they manufacture, there are surprisingly few of these factories in the UK: think in tens and hundreds, not thousands. On the chilled food front, for instance, in 2013, just 25 major chilled food companies operated from 100 highly streamlined production sites, employing around 60,000 people.

These factories supply supermarket chains that do not want the hassle of dealing with a plurality of small or medium-sized companies. With the exception of Morrisons, which is unusual in that it owns its own dedicated meat processing facilities, UK chains prefer not to get hands-on with the products they sell. Although 95% of the chilled prepared food Britain eats is sold under a retailer's brand, supermarket chains do not own the factories churning out the food and drink that bears their names. Instead, they devolve that expense, responsibility and potential risk to third-party suppliers who work at arm's length, according to the chain's specification.

In order to squeeze economies of scale from their investment, food manufacturers need to be turning out products on a fairly constant basis to make good on their outlay and investment. Time is money. Stop-start processing plants without a full production schedule don't make commercial sense, so these enterprises commonly supply not one, but several supermarket chains, to attain that critical volume. One shift, it will be Sainsbury's ready-to-grill kebabs gliding along the assembly line, the next, meatballs for Tesco, or chicken pies for Asda. Even those processed foods that are sold as familiar household brands – as opposed to supermarket own-label – are commonly manufactured by a company other than the one with its well-recognised name on the box.

This is why third-party factories have innocuous, neutral names that give little or no clue as to the nature of the enterprise. If you drive past them, they look anonymous and blank, like vast storage units. Unlike the characterful brick and stone factories that still remain from Victorian times, they have no windows.

Inside, their employees work long, demanding shifts: 12 hours isn't unusual, sometimes night shifts. They tend to be young, and driven by a very strong work ethos, the kind of people who are prepared to take any job that's going, seeing it as a stepping stone on the road to eventual financial betterment. Typically, some 90 per cent of the staff come from Eastern Europe and the Baltic States. In one workplace canteen I visited, the cook was Polish, making a daily bigos, Poland's favourite cabbage and sausage stew.

Except for the odd tantalising glimpse of the external world from the canteen windows, these people work in artificial light, in a factory world. And outsiders most certainly cannot see in, a necessary measure to guard secret recipes and commercial confidentiality, we're told.

So although these factories provide households up and down the land with billions of portions of processed food – half a million kebabs on just one day would not be unusual for a busy meat processing site – most of us haven't a clue what these mammoth population-feeding units look like inside. They don't run Doors Open Days, and any visitor, prearranged or otherwise, will be greeted by a uniformed guard, and a security barrier. Their unwritten motto? Transparency ain't us. It's not like the old days, when primary teachers would take classes to see a dairy farm and bottling plant so they could work up a cute little Day in the Life of a Pinta project. The prevailing sentiment amongst food manufacturers is that the less we have a mental picture of how our processed food is made, the better.

This defensiveness is understandable. Would most of us feel tempted by those attractively packaged and slickly marketed convenience foods, the sort of thing we choose in seconds then slip in the microwave of an evening, if we were allowed a sneak peek into the places where they were made? Not greatly, I'd wager. As for working there, they would definitely be one of the last places in the world that most people would ever want a job.

'You see, we're just a scaled-up version of a domestic kitchen', one enthusiastic boss assured me as he showed me round his pride-and-joy ready meals factory. Another executive looked me in the eye and told me with apparent conviction, and perhaps a hint of nervousness, that his meat processing plant was 'just like a biggish kitchen'. I nodded politely, but I didn't get the analogy: it's a food processor's fairy tale with all the scary bits edited out.

Food manufacturers have created a body of lore and legend around their products that sounds tremendously comforting. 'Recipes for these foods are gathered from all over the world and are created by chefs who are passionate about what they do', says the Chilled Foods Association. 'They [chefs] also like working with fresh ingredients and being involved right from the start – from initial concept to final food. They get their inspiration from different sources. Travel and cookery books are particularly important but they all love to experiment and research new ideas. Many chilled foods are hand-made in basically the same way as in the restaurant kitchen or in the home, so being able to create virtually any type of food is considered very satisfying.'

But whether they are geared up to manufacture crisps, frozen fish fingers, tinned fish, dried cereals, cheese slices, Rice Krispies®, or ready-to-microwave party canapés, factories don't look, or feel, anything like a kitchen, even of the industrial catering sort. They more resemble car plants and oil refineries, or even the missile-launching pad at the end of *Dr No*, where James Bond sabotages the efforts of a small army of operatives, lost and almost robotic-looking within the bulk of their protective clothing.

Without a detailed, highly technical explanation, or a degree in engineering, chemical engineering, microelectronics, microbiology or food technology, most of us would find it extremely hard to see any parallels with domestic food production in these cavernous factories, because there are precious few sensual or visual cues. It's not at all like those appetite-whetting TV adverts for pasta sauces, fish fingers, and other processed foods that show 'our chefs' in homely yet aspirational kitchens, surrounded by sensual displays of fresh, whole ingredients. It is most certainly not a dream job of browsing through recipe books and playing around with the world's finest and freshest ingredients. In fact, it is actually relatively rare to see anything that looks much like food as we know it in these factories, and when you do, it will most likely be swathed in strong plastic, in giant tins and cartons, or packed in cardboard boxes and stored in a freezer.

Most cooks, even hardened professional chefs and caterers with experience of institutions such as prisons and hospitals, would find this environment unfamiliar and baulk at working there for a day, let alone for a lifetime. Many of the individual industrially proportioned units of equipment would fill a generous-sized sitting room. Grouped together, they could easily occupy the ground space of a football pitch and the height of a motorway petrol station forecourt.

These factories are laid out in one seamless, highly efficient assembly-line process, designed according to a flow diagram to create the sequence of steps and tasks in the manufacturing process. Depending on the company's product lines, equipment can include spiral chillers, dehumidifiers, injectors, extruders, steam-jacketed kettles, centrifugal screeners, swept surface coolers, hoppers, sifters, oil conditioners, Stephan mixers, colloid mills, steam infusion and plate exchanger cookers, batch fryers, spray dryers, horizontal conveyor dryers, flash-cooling pumps, oven bands, freezer belts, horizontal agitators, batch and continuous lines, make-up lines, continuous mixers, high shear mixers, evaporators, and a whole apparatus of other kit that bears absolutely no resemblance to any home cook's appliances and batterie de cuisine.

The equivalent here of a domestic saucepan is a steaming vat that would require a window cleaner's ladder to look into, one with dimensions large enough to swallow up several Mafia informers at a time. Equipment clunks, spurts, grinds, squeezes, divides, stacks, minces, bakes, sucks, checks, injects, detects, chills, blasts, shapes, ploughs, agitates, steams, dries, forms, codes, freezes, defrosts, microwaves, churns, paddles, calibrates, signals, bleeps, hums, rolls, vibrates, and cools. Sauces are cooked by the ton then spewed out onto other food components that are cooked on a conveyor belt. One ready meals company is proud to say that its factory manufactures ten tons of chicken tikka a day.

The noise produced by these gargantuan pieces of plant is deafening. There's no way that you'll be humming along to Radio 2, or chatting with colleagues on the production line to help make the shift go by faster. There's no possibility of any camaraderie here. Instead, if you've any sense, you'll do what you can to protect your hearing and wear your company-provided ear plugs, then retreat for hours at a time into your own isolated, private world of thoughts, dreaming perhaps of being promoted to a better post, or finding another job doing something else entirely, until it's time for a break.

And you will need to become accustomed to working in extreme temperatures. Apart from the warmer slaughter-house and cooking stages, the ambient temperature in most zones of food factories is bitingly raw and cold, conditions that chill you down to the bone marrow. Anyone who works here will have to show endurance and stamina, and hopefully be in possession of a very robust immune system. If you tend to get a cold whenever you get chilled, you won't last long. You will also need to get accustomed to the smells. The faintly bloody smell you might find in a traditional high street butcher is one thing, but that fleshy odour, scaled up and intensified on an amplified scale because of the high through-put of carcasses, is another. If you work in a factory specialis-ing in crisps, fried breaded and battered foods, chips, or 'hand-held' snacks such as crisps and corn chips, you will come out smelling like the products you make; the fatty whiff hangs in your hair. The most off-putting smell that assailed me was in a ready meals factory, where the atmosphere was filled with the sweet, cloying scent of gloopy, viscous tomato sauce and starchy, sticky béchamel with a fragrance reminis-cent of regurgitated baby milk. Maybe people who work there stop noticing it after a while. I hope so. Working in food processing facilities is hard graft in so many ways, so it is hardly surprising that a high staff turnover and high rates of sickness absence are par for the course, or that many major plants are consistently understaffed and rely on agencies to fill the gaps. The use of temporary agency labour is common-place throughout the food industry, particularly to cover peaks in demand: the run-up to Christmas, for instance.

The less experienced jobs in food processing are so unremittingly monotonous, repetitive and unrewarding that they must surely depress the spirits and elevate stress levels. Who wants to spend 12 hours a day arranging meatballs as though they were boxes of chocolates, or checking that there are four cubes of meat in every portion of chicken casserole, according to the product specification? But some food processing jobs are highly skilled. Although most people would consider it the most grizzly, hellish job in the world, the slaughterhouse men who take a dead whole carcass and 'dissemble' it – that's breaking it down into its main parts, stripping back the skin and hide, vacuuming out spinal cord, splicing heads in two, removing tendons and hoofs, brains, pancreas, kidneys, suet, collecting ears and thymus, emptying colons, examining lymph nodes, separating guts, cutting out the major bones, pulling off membranes, de-gristling and segregating everything that hasn't a food or other use to produce fore- and hind-quarters for further butchery – are consummate experts.

Those whom I have seen working on the carcass 'dissembly' line move at a fierce pace: a state-of-the-art abattoir can break down a whole cow into quarters and bag them, in 40 minutes. There, staff typically operate non-stop for three and a half hours at a time in a hot, steamy, visceral atmosphere, demonstrating a certainty and adroitness that comes from experience. In food processing terms, they are well paid, because they have to concentrate intently, each and every second, on what they are doing.

Their task requires training, physical strength, endurance, precision knife skills, excellent hand-to-eye coordination, and a developed understanding of anatomy. Their brains need to be engaged every second. A slip of the knife, a moment's lapse of attention, and a gory catalogue of accidents is waiting to happen. The jobs of these slaughtermen are repetitive, but they aren't dull or unintelligent any more than that of the craft jeweller or clockmaker, who peers into the innards of watches all day, making minute adjustments and repairs.

For their part, the food-factory boss men, who have nice, bright, clean offices with lots of windows, upstairs, or in another building, talk not of 'food', but of 'product'. The word 'cooking' doesn't come into it; they use the more honest term: 'manufacture'. Industry top brass refers not to ingredients, but 'food ingredient technology' and 'food ingredients systems'. Their vocabulary speaks volumes about how companies view the job in hand.

Food processing executives have a long list of daily hygiene and food safety concerns, because danger is omnipresent in the industrial food system. Metal detection, for instance, requires an entire strategy, part of the ongoing military campaign to prevent any uninvited foreign object from getting into your microwaveable meal, sandwich or prepared salad. With so many complex, intricate pieces of industrial equipment in use, there is always a very real possibility that a screw, nut or some other piece of equipment drops into your macaroni cheese. Allergens are another constant bugbear. A trace of soya or peanut where it ought not to be, and a whole day's production is scuppered.

Given the high risk inherent in industrial-scale food manufacture, record-keeping is critical. Every piece of equipment and ingredient must come with a paper trail to vouch for its origins and safety. The managers below the boss men have internal audits – essentially box-ticking exercises – coming out of their ears. They supervise elaborate coding schemes to ensure that each and every product that goes through the production process is traceable back to a specific batch, grade and type, made at a specific time of day. That's no mean effort: a ready meals factory can be churning out 250,000 individual servings a day, made up of 60 or 70 different products, using ten different assembly lines. One leading ready meals manufacturer, for instance, boasts that it makes 2.5 million ready meals a week.

When large industrial plants are churning out such a product volume, you might think that public health authorities would drop in at intervals to check that everything is up to scratch. That happens, but not as frequently as you might assume. Official statistics show, for example, that more than 55 per cent of all registered UK food establishments did not receive a local authority health inspection or audit in the year April 2012 to March 2013. Julia Long, the Unite union's national officer for the food sector, sums up this situation as follows:

> Food processing is one of our fastest-growing industries, employing hundreds of thousands of workers. The industry needs an inspection regime that respects this and understands that public safety and confidence are paramount. At the moment, thanks to the running down of the service, a business can look forward to an inspection only once in a blue moon.

Instead, the food industry is largely left to monitor its own food hygiene and safety procedures, using a system known as HACCP: Hazard Analysis and Critical Control Point. This involves continuously monitoring every 'critical control point' where a likely hazard might arise – food poisoning bacteria, cross-contamination, and more – and keeping copious trails of paperwork to show that all possible checks have been vigilantly carried out. The emphasis in food chain regulation these days is on internal prevention, not external, independent inspection.

And yet, a lot can go wrong quickly when you manufacture convenience food at considerable speed on an industrial scale, and if it does, the consequences are extremely serious. If you're talking food poisoning, the affected batch will have been loaded onto lorries, trucked to supermarket distribution centres, and laid out on shelves, making thousands of people ill within hours, in which case, there will be hell to pay. If the problem is rogue allergens, manufacturers will have to meet the considerable cost of a product recall. The penalties that can be imposed on them by retailers are severe, everything from being fined to losing the business.

The authorities will become involved, which is something of an embarrassment for the retailer, with knock-on consequences for the manufacturer. It could mean a 'trade recall', the recovery of the product from distribution centres, wholesalers, hospitals, restaurants, other major catering establishments, as well as other food processors, and/or it might also lead to a 'consumer recall', a complete withdrawal of the products from retail outlets. Product recall notices will have to be displayed in stores, along the lines of 'If you have bought one of the products listed above, do not eat it. Instead, return it to the store it was bought from for a full refund or contact customer services'. Hundreds of thousands of refunds will have to be paid out.

Yet despite the dire consequences manufacturers face when their production goes wrong, recalls are surprisingly common in the UK. Barely a week goes by without one. Sometimes there are several recalls in one day. Take, for instance, 25 February 2014, when the Food Standards Agency (FSA) issued the following alert:

> Sainsbury's has recalled its 'by Sainsbury's' Frozen Sticky Toffee Sponge Pudding, because the product may contain small pieces of metal.

This communication was swiftly followed by another:

> Marks & Spencer has withdrawn its Lightly Dusted Salt and Pepper British Chicken Fillets because a small number of packs contain egg, which is not mentioned on the label. This makes the product a possible health risk for anyone who is allergic or has an intolerance to egg.

And yet another:

> Sainsbury's has withdrawn all packs of Sainsbury's Taste the Difference Roasted Chestnut, Toasted Hazelnut & Thyme Stuffing because the product may contain traces of peanut due to cross contamination during manufacturing. This is not mentioned on the label making the product a possible health risk for anyone who is allergic to peanuts.

Presence of allergens is by far the most common reason for product recalls, but why is this? Obsessed with being cost-effective, many food processors operate the food factory equivalent of hot-desking by redeploying the same plant equipment and assembly line, often in the course of a day, to make several different products. So a factory will be set up to handle a range of foods of one production type. For instance, a factory geared up for continuous production of smooth products with small particles can handle soups, sauces, desserts, baby food purées, fruit and tomato preparations. One with a continuous instant and dehydrated line is custom built to manufacture things like packet soups, gravy granules and stock powders.

Whatever the factory specialism, every last bit of equipment should be thoroughly cleaned and sanitised between batches of different products so that each new batch starts from a clean slate, but the frequency and regularity of allergen recalls shows that this is not always the case. 'Nut Trace Contamination' (NTC) warnings on processed foods that read 'may contain nuts/nut traces' or 'produced in a factory using nuts', are ostensibly aimed at people who suffer from nut allergies. In extreme cases, they can develop a severe, life-threatening reaction, anaphylaxis. However, the ubiquity of NTC warnings on manufactured products hints at the underlying problem of controlling factory food. Such warnings are an admission of defeat, an acknowledgement that because of the sheer complication and complexity of the factory equipment, and the speed of production, manufacturers do not have, and can never have, total control of what ends up in their food. In fact, preventing cross-contamination, be that from peanuts or any other ingredient, is quite beyond them.

Unless you suffer from nut allergies – in which case it's a matter of life and death, you may have only been mildly perplexed by the appearance of NTC warnings on products where nuts aren't listed as an ingredient. Why would there be nuts in your pitta bread, chilli con carne seasoning mix, or your ready-to-heat Thai vegetable soup, after all? When the FSA researched consumers' views of NTC warnings, people told them in no uncertain terms that they were unclear as to their meaning. 'The equivocal nature of the phrases had been universally resented by respondents', the FSA reported. Furthermore, they were 'seen as an insurance policy for manufacturers'. That conclusion is shrewd. Food manufacturers do spend a lot of time watching their backs and limiting their liability precisely because they are in a high-risk business.

Whether it's a case of allergens, contamination with food poisoning bugs, or rotting food, any such 'production faults' (as they are known in the industry) will very likely hit several seemingly distinct and separate lines simultaneously. When one such factory supplying Tesco was informed that some rice in packs had become mouldy, for example, the FSA had to issue a product recall information notice on all batches of no less than eight ready meals: chicken jalfrezi, Szechuan chicken, chilli con carne, chicken tikka masala, beef in black bean sauce, sweet and sour chicken, chicken korma and balti vegetable curry. The sheer scale and productivity of the manufacturing enterprise also clocks up risk: a typical factory might be 'cooking' 2,000 portions of rice at a time in the same machine. So when a problem arises on the production line, it affects millions of portions of food in no time at all.

Are these mammoth food factories really just scaled-up versions of a domestic kitchen, as manufacturers would lead us to believe? If consumers of their products had an accurate mental picture of how their products were made, they could arbitrate on this point by casting an informed vote. But in the modern convenience food system, production is strictly out of sight and out of mind. Food retailers prefer us to focus on more attractive things – their adverts, the luscious marketing images on the packaging, the special offers and promotions, anything, in fact, other than what actually happens down on the factory floor. And having gained access to this strange and unsettling world for myself, I'd say that was an extremely wise policy.

3

Clean label

Food manufacturers have embarked on a major exercise designed to quell our fears about the composition of their products. They were forced into it. Food investigations provide regular editorial meat for the media. Millions of us read books and articles and watch exposés on how the food we eat is produced, setting up nagging worries.

Sensitised by scare and scandal, more of us now approach processed food with a sceptical eye. We scan labels for E numbers, the European Union's code for substances used as additives, because we see them as flashing red alerts for nutritionally compromised, low-grade industrial food. As one food industry commentator put it, 'E numbers have a very high "label-polluting" effect'. We home in on ingredients and additives with long chemical names. What on earth is carboxymethylcellulose, or mono- and diacetyl tartaric esters of mono- and diglycerides of fatty acids, we wonder, and an increasing number of us are deeply suspicious of foods that contain them.

A growing citizen army wants to eat real food, and seeks out what's come to be known as the 'kitchen-cupboard' guarantee: if you wouldn't use mystery ingredients X, Y and Z in your own cooking, why on earth would you eat them in ready-made food? As one food processing executive explains: 'One of the problems we face is people's confidence in chemicals. Chemicals is [sic] seen as a nasty word.'

For decades, the chemical industry tried to put a lid on this grassroots revolt by arming food manufacturers and retailers with a pat little keep-calm-and-carry-on script. Here, in the words of the International Food Additives Council, a trade association representing the interests of food additive and ingredient producers, is how it goes:

> With well over 2,300 food additives currently approved for use, it would be staggering to list the components of each of these substances. However, every additive – like every food we consume – no matter what its source or intended purpose, is composed of chemicals. Everything, including the clothes we wear, the cars we drive, the foods we eat, even our own bodies, is made up of chemicals.

The sub-text here, just in case you had missed it, is that those of us who worry about additives and inscrutable industrial ingredients are scientific incompetents, who, if we really understood the science, wouldn't be in the least bit alarmed. The argument is further elaborated in a dogged attempt to put an end to the persistent, seditious line of thought that processed food is qualitatively different from natural food:

> There is much discussion regarding 'natural' and 'synthetic' chemicals. Many of those synthesised in the laboratory are also found naturally occurring in foods. Chemicals are chemicals; the distinction between a 'natural' and

> 'synthetic' chemical is itself artificial. The molecular structure of each is exactly the same and the human body does not discriminate based upon the source. For example, sugar found in sugar cane (sucrose) is no different in composition and function than refined sugar. Similarly, citric acid produced commercially by enzymatic fermentation, is the same naturally occurring chemical that makes lemons tart. To say one chemical is safer than another because of its origin simply does not make sense.

Note the implication in that final phrase: anyone who is suspicious of processed food is an irrational, confused hysteric.

How disappointing it must be for the companies that have invested so much time and effort in disseminating this message to see that it simply hasn't been believed. Despite their concerted efforts to rubbish public concerns about the additives in processed food, they just won't go away. Realists in the food industry now accept this is the case, as this industry spokesman explains:

> We know that consumers want a return to familiar ingredients and in recent years, terms such as 'natural', 'authentic', 'preservative-free' and 'additive-free' have proliferated on the packaging of food products in Europe. These clearly portray the consumer's desire to return to simple, less-processed ingredients which are familiar to everyone, and the rejection of additives. For agri-food companies, claiming 100% natural products, and crusading against additives, leads to success in Europe.

It's the same story worldwide. When the US Whole Foods Market chain issued a roll call of ingredients that it would not permit in any of the products it sold, this 'Unacceptable Ingredients for Food' list sent shock waves through the global food industry. This list currently runs to over 70 additives and obscure industrial ingredients, from acesulfame K, ammonium chloride and azodicarbonamide, to tert-butylhydroquinone, tetrasodium EDTA and vanillin, and it is added to from time to time as controversial ingredients shoot up the public agenda. In the case of high fructose corn syrup, for instance, a sweetener that is increasingly in the frame as a key driver of the US obesity epidemic, Whole Foods Market gave its suppliers until the end of 2010 to reformulate and remove it from all products destined for its stores.

Whole Foods Market, of course, is often stereotyped as catering for the worried wealthy, but every other food retailer now knows that perceived naturalness is a very effective shortcut to what's known as 'premiumisation', that is, getting your customers to believe that your products are good quality. As one observer of food industry trends explains, 'many [product] formulators do turn to the list of unacceptable ingredients published by Whole Foods'.

Now that once stalwart additives and ingredients have their names up there in flashing red lights, food manufacturers have a major headache. They have come to rely on flavourings and obscure sweeteners to replace the natural tastes in food that industrial processing destroys. They have depended on fake colours to make over-processed, degraded beige-brown food look more appealing. They have needed preservatives and antioxidants to extend shelf life. Without these, and all the other weapons in its trusty armoury – emulsifiers, stabilisers, sequestrants, gelling agents, thickeners, anti-foaming agents, bulking agents, carriers and carrier solvents, emulsifying salts, firming agents, flavour enhancers, flour-treatment agents, foaming agents, glazing agents, humectants, propellants, raising agents, flavour carriers and binders – the modern processed food industry is drained of its life blood.

So under pressure to clean up their act, many food manufacturers have latched on to the emerging concept of 'clean label'. In the last decade, this is the big idea that has moved from the health-store margins of the food industry to grip the mainstream. The term has no legal definition, but in the industry, 'clean label' is widely taken to mean that the *ancien régime* of food additives, with all its negative connotations, has been replaced or removed, that the ingredient listing is simple, that is, made up of recognisable ingredients that do not sound chemical or artificial, and that the product has been processed 'using traditional techniques that are understood by consumers and not perceived as being artificial'. As the director of one market research company put it, the word 'natural' 'works as a heuristic to shoppers, a shortcut to a product being good for them, something they'd be happy to give their children'.

Some companies have taken up the clean label concept to reformulate their products in a genuine, wholehearted way, replacing ingredients and additives that raise health or quality concerns with substitutes that are generally thought to be less problematic. Other companies, however, unconvinced that they can pass on the cost of radical reformulation to food retailers and consumers, have turned to a novel range of substances that allow them to present a much more scrubbed and rosy face to the public, without incurring excessive cost. In their hands, clean labelling has become an exercise that dispenses with the services of the food industry's dirty dozens, and introduces us to an initially more wholesome and healthy-looking bunch of new friends.

The challenge faced by companies under pressure to reformulate products has been to find alternative ingredients that can perform the same functions as the old 'nasties' – that is, they must cost less than the natural equivalent, have a good shelf life and be easy to process – but can be described in a much more appetising way. In this endeavour, food manufacturers look to a plethora of global ingredient supply companies that understand their technical needs and provide clean label solutions to the food manufacturer's dirty little label problems. In the industry's own terminology, these solutions aim to square the consumer's yearning for naturalness with the manufacturer's need for 'functionality'. In practical terms, what this means is that even if you are a thoughtful eater, someone who diligently inspects product labels, food manufacturers are always one step ahead of you. In fact, if you are still fretting about E numbers, you are way behind the curve. That was food awareness reading book number one; now we are on to reading book number two.

Supposing, for example, you were standing in the supermarket eyeing up a pot of something temptingly called a 'chocolate cream dessert'. You read the ingredients: whole milk, sugar (well, there has to be some in there), cream, cocoa powder and dark chocolate (they all sound quite up-market), but then your urge to buy falters as you notice three feel-bad ingredients. The first of these is carrageenan (E407). You may or may not have read headlines reporting that this setting agent, derived from seaweed, has been linked with ulcers and gastrointestinal cancer, but even if you haven't, there's a good chance that the E number will put you off anyway. Carrageenan belongs to a group of gummy substances, including guar, agar, konjac, inulin, locust bean, acacia, xanthan, cellulose and pectin, known as hydrocolloids. It is now regarded in food industry circles as an 'ideally not' [to be included] additive.

The second of these worrying ingredients is a modified starch (E1422), or to give it its full chemical name, acetylated distarch adipate. It started off its life as a simple starch, of the kind you'd find naturally in potatoes or rice, but it has been chemically altered to increase its water-holding capacity and tolerance for the extreme temperatures and physical pressures of industrial-scale processing. Spot this, and chances are that the term 'modified' will put you off, and if it doesn't, then the bothersome E number most likely will.

The third problematical ingredient is gelatine. It's anathema to observant Muslims, Jews and vegetarians, and even secular omnivores may be wondering what this by-product of porcine hides is doing in their pudding.

Fortunately for the manufacturers of your chocolate cream dessert, there is a Plan B. They can remove all three offending items, and replace them with a more sophisticated type of 'functional flour' hydrothermally extracted from cereals, that will do the same job, but without the need for E numbers. 'Because they are flours' explains the sales pitch for one such product, 'all our ingredients produce home-made and additive-free textures with a touch of authenticity to make products stand out from the crowd ... Our functional flours have a reassuring declaration as 'wheat', 'corn' or 'rice' flour – simple ingredients familiar to everyone.'

Another possibility for cleaning up this dessert would be to use a 'co-texturiser' that would cost-effectively deliver the necessary thick and creamy indulgence factor. As the supplier of one such product puts it: 'They bring out the more subtle differences in texture that we experience in our mouths while eating, such as mouthcoating and meltaway.' Texturisers, just like modified starches, are based on highly processed, altered starch designed to withstand high-volume, high-temperature, high-pressure manufacturing, but because they are obligingly classified by food regulators as a 'functional native starch', they can be labelled simply as 'starch', with no troublesome E number at the end.

So, out come two additives and one ingredient that many people avoid, to be replaced by a single new generation ingredient, one that is opaque in its formulation – proprietary secrets, and all that – but which won't trigger consumer alarm.

With the chocolate dessert in your trolley, you find yourself at the deli counter. Fancy a dip for dunking your nachos? Possibly not, if you noticed that they contained an old-school preservative with an E number after its incomprehensible name, something such as sodium benzoate, or sorbate, nitrites, nitrates and sulfites. Not only do these sound like science lab chemicals, you might also have heard that several of them have been linked to ADD, allergies and cancer. But food manufacturers can get round your resistance by using instead a label-friendly preservative, made by fermenting corn or cane sugar with specific cultures that form organic acids and fermentation products; these have a similar bacteria-inhibiting effect. The boon here for the manufacturer is that they can be labelled as 'cultured cane/corn syrup', or 'cultured vinegar', and that sounds positively classy.

Maybe you usually buy some cold cooked meat, turkey perhaps, or ham? It's always useful for sandwiches and easy meals. Food-wise shoppers tend to be doubly vigilant while shopping in this category. Hanky-panky in the meat department always has potential to trigger a yuck reaction, and the presence of phosphates on a label is widely interpreted as an ominous sign. It provides evidence of meat that has been swollen by injecting it, or 'tumbling' it in a drum, with bulking chemicals and water. So processed meat manufacturers are increasingly turning to clean label 'phosphate replacers', sticky, binding substances derived from tapioca and other starchy foods, that do the job of retaining added water, but allow a chemical-free label. Observant shoppers might notice the presence of tapioca starch on the ingredients list, and wonder vaguely how a tropical tuber got into their sliced ham, but it sounds a whole lot more cuddly than sodium/potassium/calcium/ammonium polyphosphate E452.

Picking up some rustic-looking salami, even the most guarded shoppers might relax when they notice rosemary extract on the ingredients list. We'd love to believe that this cured meat has been lovingly aromatised with fragrant herbs. Actually, rosemary extracts are clean label substitutes for the old guard of techie-sounding antioxidants (E300-21), such as butylhydroxyanisole (BHA) and butylhydroxytoluene (BHT). Food manufacturers use them to slow down the rate at which foods go rancid, so extending their shelf life; basically, they act as preservatives.

Rosemary extracts do have an E number (E392) but manufacturers prefer to label them more poetically as 'extract of rosemary', and lose the offending E, because that way they sound like lovingly made Slow Food ingredients, especially if they are also labelled as natural or organic. Never believe for a moment that this antioxidant in your salami is there to provide an aromatic herbiness: its role is to stop the meat discolouring in air so that it retains that desirable fresh appearance for weeks.

Rosemary extracts do, at one stage of their production process, have something to do with the eponymous herb, albeit usually in its dried, rather than fresh, form. However, the herb's antioxidant chemicals (phenolic diterpenes called carnosol and carnosic acid) are isolated in an extraction procedure that 'deodorises' them, that is to say, removes any rosemary taste and smell. Extraction is done either by the supercritical fluid-extraction method, which uses carbon dioxide, or using chemical solvents. The solvents in question are hexane (derived from the fractional distillation of petroleum), ethanol (a petrol replacer from the fermentation of sugar and starch), and acetone (the flammable pungent fluid that dissolves nail varnish). Neutral-tasting rosemary extract is then sold to manufacturers, usually in the form of a brownish powder. In short, the connection that rosemary extract has with the freshly cut, green and pungent herb we know and love is considerably more remote than we might like to think.

As you make your way up and down the aisles, note how that word 'extract' increasingly features on ingredient listings; not just rosemary either, but carrot, paprika, beetroot and more. What, exactly, are they doing in your breakfast cereals, your lunchtime sandwich and your evening ready meal? Unlike rosemary, they are used as clean label colourings. Carrot extract, for instance, is popular in food manufacturing because it lends a golden hue to everything from ready-made custard and cakes to salad dressings and yogurts.

Food manufacturers can buy it in various shades, such as 'warm orange' or 'shining yellow'. The process of obtaining it starts with real carrots in some form, not necessarily fresh or whole. The natural orange colour, carotene, is extracted in a similar process to rosemary extract. If manufacturers want a dash of red colour to make their yogurt look fruitier and more berried, they can use extract of beetroot (betanin), or grapes (anthocyanins). For a brownish-red, safflower extract will do the job, or if you're after more of a cool, cosmopolitan cappuccino, there's malt extract.

Extracts sound so much nicer than that abrasive word 'colouring', and they play well with the health-conscious shopper who has picked up a few key words, such as anthocyanins, from the health pages of magazines. They come over a bit like added-value, vitality-boosting superfood compounds, something you might buy as a food supplement from a health food store, and hold a particularly strong appeal for the mother who frets about what's in her toddler's snack pack. Sometimes carrot or paprika extract is labelled as 'mixed carotenes', and that term has a glowing halo of health. After all, it has something to do with carrots, hasn't it? And we all know that vegetables are good for us. Maybe beetroot extract is actually a nifty idea from food manufacturers to help parents con their children into eating nutritious vegetables without them knowing it? Actually, that assumption couldn't be further from the truth. No extract has a nutritional profile that comes anywhere close to that of the source vegetable or fruit in its whole, raw state, because the extraction process ruins it. Furthermore, extracts are supplied to manufacturers in different forms – powder, liquid, oil, and emulsion – with other additives in the mix, such as maltodextrin and modified starch as carriers and emulsifiers, or the preservative potassium sorbate, or in a handy sugar syrup with propylene glycol, a solvent, better known for its anti-freeze effect. Nice idea though it is, extracts make absolutely no contribution to your five-a-day.

If extracts won't do the trick, another handy new form of colouring that doesn't sound like colouring sneaks on to the label in the form of micronised powders. These are plant foods dried and pulverised into particles that are only a few microns in diameter. Broccoli powder provides green, cranberry powder provides red and, as with extracts, the mention of healthy fruit or vegetables will help make even a packet of sweets look as if it is positively brimming with goodness.

As clean label extracts and powders colonise product labels, one additive with bad PR that is less and less to be seen is E150 caramel, formerly food manufacturers' go-to prop for imbuing products with sweet flavour and brown colour. It is being replaced with clean label 'burnt caramelised sugar', 'caramelised sugar syrup', 'burnt sugar syrup' and 'caramelised sugar'. Although these substances give a similar effect to unpopular old E150, they aren't classed as food additives, but as ingredients, so no E number is required. Even when they are being used purely for food colouring purposes, they need only be declared as 'plain caramel', words that evoke the image of something you'd make at home for a toothsome crème caramel. As one supplier explains:

> Our caramelised sugar syrups offer a range of sweet to burnt notes, compatibility with caramel colors, high-alcohol solubility in spirits and liqueurs, processing stability in salt, flavor enhancer capabilities, natural products oppor-

> tunities, clean-label benefits; may be labeled as 'sugar'. Caramelised sugar syrups provide both flavor and color in one blend.

Weighing up the products on sale in the bakery department – will it be this loaf or those rolls? – the mention of emulsifiers such as soy lecithin, or mono- and diglycerides of fatty acids (E471), might not do much to recommend a product to you. After all, they don't figure in any home baker's recipe. Thinking clean label, manufacturers can switch to rice extract made by modifying rice bran with protease enzymes; these perform the same task of binding oil and water in the dough. The word enzyme would not have to appear on the ingredients listing; a more label-friendly 'rice extract' would suffice. A further bonus, as the maker of one such rice product says, is that such ingredients 'can improve a manufacturer's bottom line by eliminating or reducing many common production problems'. Specifically, 'the cost saving is immediate by allowing formulations to contain more water, reducing the use of costlier ingredients, improving output and reducing breakage'. However much consumers are preoccupied with trying to keep down their food bills, rest assured, food manufacturers are every bit as keenly focused on reducing theirs.

Still not sure what you're going to eat for dinner? Why not backtrack to the ready-meal aisle and pick up something instant and tasty – a chicken noodle dish, perhaps, maybe a pizza. If you noticed that it contained an amino acid, such as L-cysteine E910, your enthusiasm might wane, especially if you were a clued-up vegan who happens to know that this additive can be derived from animal and human hair. L-cysteine has been an extremely useful additive for food manufacturers. In your pizza, it acts as a dough 'conditioner' (strengthener). In your chicken noodles, it brings a meaty, savoury flavour to the table. But its presence on a label is something of an embarrassment to processing companies these days, so a range of new-wave yeast extracts is increasingly replacing it. One supplier of such extracts markets its products to food manufacturers as follows:

> This range offers you a variety of pre-composed, ready-to-use products that provide the same intensity as our classical process flavors ... but ... are labeled as all-natural. Ingredients are available in chicken and beef flavor, with roasted or boiled varieties, as well as white meat and dark roast.

These hi-tech yeast extracts equip manufacturers with the range of meaty, caramelised, barbecued, brothy, roasted 'middle block flavours' they are accustomed to working with. There are quite a few to choose from, depending on the nature of the food in question, and the impact required. A manufacturer can add a little touch of an extract that brings a 'brothy, white meaty, sweet umami enhancement', or ramp up the flavour with another that promises 'natural roast sulphury chicken aroma notes'. Both can be labelled as 'yeast extract' without any mention that they are being used as flavourings. That's quite a boon to manufacturers, because yeast extracts have a healthy image, particularly amongst vegetarians, as a rich source of B vitamins. Less well known is the fact that yeast extract has a high concentration of the amino acid glutamate, from which monosodium glutamate – better known as MSG, one of the most shunned additives – is derived. In other words, yeast extract is just another member of the meaty, muscular, flavour-enhancing glutamate clan. A case of plus ça change, plus c'est la même chose, by any chance?

As you wend your way up and down supermarket aisles these days, it is certainly becoming easier to let your guard drop. Food manufacturers now seem to understand our concerns and increasingly speak to us in a coaxing language we want to hear. They offer us products that appear to be reformed, reconstructed, improved versions of their predecessors. These come plastered with tick lists and upbeat front-of-pack claims, and when we turn them over, their ingredients listings seem relatively short and sweet. Descriptions such as 'natural' and 'additive-free' get us to suspend our disbelief and keep buying; they trigger a positive why-bother-cooking sentiment in us. As one executive in a leading ingredients supply company put it: 'Ingredients that *give the impression* [my emphasis] that they originated in a grandmother's kitchen and have not been processed too harshly are of great appeal to consumers.'

Whether the clean label campaign is indeed a heart and soul effort by food manufacturers to respond to our desire for more wholesome, less mucked around with food, or just a self-interested substitution exercise, is a matter of opinion. Additives and ingredients presented as benign one day have a habit of looking less innocent the next as we learn more about the means by which they were created, and how they affect our health. In the meantime, it is worth noting that clean label is not causing assembly lines to grind to a halt, use-by dates to shorten, or production rates to dwindle. Neither is there any evidence that food manufacturers are using greater quantities of the real, natural ingredients that consumers want to eat. Thus far, clean label looks less like a thorough spring clean of factory food than a superficial tidy-up, with the most embarrassing mess stuffed in the cupboard behind a firmly shut door, where hopefully no-one will notice it.

4
At the food makers' market

Where do the companies that manufacture our processed food do their shopping? The European marketplace for this business is an annual trade show called Food Ingredients. Under one roof, over three days, this exhibition hosts the world's most important gathering of ingredient suppliers, distributors and buyers. Think of it as the food manufacturer's equivalent of an arms fair.

At Food Ingredients, the buyers, representatives of companies that make our ready meals and convenience foods, meet sellers with imposing job titles – Global Procurement Ingredients Director, European Lead Buyer and Innovation Partner, R&D Product Developer, Ingredient Specification Technologist, Product and Application Development Manager, Formulation Project Leader – who present them with the 'personalised solutions they need to grow and nurture their business'.

Food Ingredients represents the beating heart of the modern food industry, showcasing its very latest innovations and trends, and its dialogue is thoroughly international. In 2011, when it was held in Paris, over 23,000 visitors attended from 154 countries – industry movers and shakers who collectively represented an ingredient buying power of €4 billion.

Consistent with the industry view that the general public is best given only the sketchiest notion of what goes on behind the scenes of food processing, Food Ingredients events aren't open to the general public. Anyone who tries to register has to show that they work in food manufacturing but, using a fake ID, I managed to register for Food Ingredients 2013. It was housed in the vast, eerie expanses of Frankfurt's Blade Runner-like Festhalle Messe, a fitting venue that mirrors the sheer scale of modern food manufacturing.

For those who love to cook and eat, food trade exhibitions are sometimes alienating, disillusioning experiences, a through-the-keyhole insight into aspects of food production you'd rather not know about, but Food Ingredients had a surreal quality all of its own. I wasn't greeted by the smell of food, and hardly anything on display much resembled it. While exhibitors at most food exhibitions are often keen for you to taste their products, at Food Ingredients, few of the stand-holders had anything instantly edible to offer. That's possibly something to do with the fact that their potential customers, while prepared to buy the products on display for manufacturing, don't much fancy eating them.

And even the foods at those stands that did want visitors to taste something weren't all that they seemed. Canapé-style cubes of white cheese dusted with herbs and spices sat under a bistro-style blackboard that nonchalantly read 'Feta, with Glucono-Delta-Lactone'; the latter ingredient is, apparently, a 'cyclic ester of gluconic acid' that acts as an acidifier, thus prolonging shelf life. A pastry chef in gleaming whites was rounding off his live demonstration by offering sample petit fours to the buyers who had gathered. His dainty heart- and diamond-shaped cakes were dead ringers for those neat layers of sponge, glossy fruit jelly, foamy cream and chocolate you'd see in the window of a classy patisserie, but were made entirely without eggs, butter or cream, thanks to the crafty substitution of potato protein isolate. This revolutionary ingredient is 'tailored to the required functionality: foaming, emulsifying, or gelling' and provides 'the volume, texture, stability and mouthfeel' we look for in classic cakes, baked with traditional ingredients.

Many exhibitors had striking visual displays, arranged like installations at an art gallery. Gleaming glass shelves were back-lit to show off a rainbow of super-sized phials of liquids so bright with colouring, they might be neon. Plates of various powders, shaped into pyramids, were artistically stacked on elegant Perspex stands bearing enigmatic labels, such as 'texturised soy protein: minced ham colour', or displayed in cabinets, as though they were exhibits in a museum.

Walls were given over to geometric displays of powdery substances, from white, through beige and brown to orange in hue, each bearing an alphanumeric code, and glowing white, yet cryptic captions that read 'pork skin products', 'beef products', or similar. One porthole-sized convex glass round housed a liquid that captured the hue of harbour water on a dark night, another framed a solitary blueberry muffin. I had to keep reminding myself that this wasn't some art college end-of-term show though, because these intriguing objects were, according to the explanatory signage, 'solutions for coating, glazing, polishing, releasing, emulsifying'. Still unsure what, exactly, I was looking at, the further information 'flavour vehicles', 'MCT oils' and 'pan oil' didn't hugely enlighten me.

Seeing a plate of puce-striped, chocolate-coated granola bars centre stage in a glass case, my initial reaction was that some avant-garde artist was making an ironic comment on modern life, like Carl André's controversial floor of bricks at the Tate Gallery. But then I read the notice: 'cereal bar with compound coating: oil-dispersible technology of 'plain' caramel colour and beetroot red', and realised that everyone else was taking them deadly seriously.

Perhaps the most beautifully curated artefacts on display were vases containing glowing orange liquids – some cloudy, some crystal clear – for colouring fruit juices. One looked particularly spectacular, like a lava lamp with ghostly threads of gossamer-like material suspended evenly in it. These were 'orange cells': they come in handy, apparently, for making those cartons of juice composed of pasteurised orange concentrate and water look as though they contain some freshly squeezed juice.

In the absence of any sight or smell to whet the appetite, a lay visitor to Food Ingredients, one who was not part of the food manufacturing fraternity, might feel the need to double check that they were indeed at a food exhibition. For Food Ingredients is so clearly the domain of a technocracy of engineers and scientists, people whose natural environment is the laboratory and the factory, not the kitchen, the farm or the field, people who share the assumption that everything nature can do, man can do so much better, and more profitably.

The broad business interest portfolio of the companies exhibiting at Food Ingredients was disconcerting. For instance, the Swiss company DKSH, whose sales pitch is 'performance materials, concepts and ingredients for the confectionery and bakery industry', described itself as 'a leading speciality chemicals and ingredients supplier'. Its business interests span 'speciality chemicals, food and beverage industry, pharmaceutical industry, and the personal care industry'.

Omya, which seemed proud to be based in Hamburg because it is 'the largest chemical trading place in the world', announced itself as 'a leading global chemical distributor and producer of industrial minerals'. The company reeled off its list of markets as food, pet food, oleochemicals, cosmetics, personal care, detergents, cleaners, papers, adhesives, construction, plastics, and industrial chemicals. Omya was at Food Ingredients selling products as diverse as granular onion powder, monosodium glutamate and phosphoric acid.

Corbion, a 'global market leader in lactic acid, lactic acid derivatives, and a leading company in functional blends containing enzymes, emulsifiers, minerals and vitamins' pointed out that its products have applications not only in bakery and meat, but also in 'pharmaceuticals and medical devices, home and personal care, packaging, automotive, coatings and coating resins'.

Helm AG introduced itself as 'one of the world's biggest chemical marketing companies'. It has sales offices in more than 30 countries across the globe, and a product portfolio that includes chemicals, 'crop protection' (pesticides), pharmaceuticals and medical products, animal and human nutrition, and fertiliser. It appears to be a big name in artificial sweeteners, with products such as Acesulfame K, Cyclamate and Aspartame.

Wacker, from Munich, trumpeted that it is 'one of the world's leading and most research-intensive chemical companies'; no exaggeration there, given that in 2008 its sales totalled €4.3 billion. It too had a catholic range of products, which it catalogued as 'silicones, binders and polymer additives for diverse industrial sectors to bio-engineered pharmaceutical actives and hyperpure silicon for semi-conductor and solar applications'.

At Food Ingredients, I rapidly realised that for big companies with a finger in many business pies, food processing is just another revenue stream. They experience no cognitive dissonance in providing components not only for your ready meal, but also for your fly spray, air freshener, shower sealant, deodorant, computer casing, scratch-resistant car coating, paint and glue. But as a food manufacturing outsider, this queasy juxtaposition of the industrial and the edible comes as a sobering shock.

You don't have to be at Food Ingredients for any time at all to pick up the central marketing message of companies selling their wares to food manufacturers. The strapline for a product called Butter Buds®, described by its makers as 'an enzyme-modified encapsulated butter flavour that has as much as 400 times the flavor intensity of butter', summed it up in six words: 'When technology meets nature, you save'. And just in case that was too airy-fairy, the small print spelled it out: 'Using Butter Buds saves you money, resulting in a healthier profit margin'. Or plainer still: 'Butter Buds helps you cut costs'.

In fact, as I walked round the exhibition, it was apparent that the main point of Food Ingredients is to sell food manufacturers wonder products that allow them to reduce their spend on more costly, real ingredients. The show is a bazaar stacked with merchandise that will be 'cost-effective at low dosages', 'generate cost savings', 'improve profit margins and yields' and allow for 'cost optimisation'. In the words of All in All, an Irish company that supplies brines, binders and stabilisers for comminuted (processed) meats and rotisserie chicken: 'Why buy ingredients when you can buy solutions?'

'Solutions', of course, is a buzzword in food manufacturing, the thinking being that natural, unprocessed food is just one big headache, loads of hassle and too much expense. Accept this premise, and it's obvious that any financially prudent manufacturer needs customised adaptations of natural food, 'functional' components designed for their production process.

Manufacturers look to the companies that supply them to collaborate, or in industry speak, to 'co-create' and design the processed foods that line our shelves. Given the ever-growing range of such ingredients with very specific physical characteristics, modern food manufacturing is potentially a quagmire of technical complexity. In this industry, few ingredients are totally straightforward. A seasoning is rarely just a spice, more often it is part of a 'seasoning system' or 'coating system'. Meat is hardly ever meat as a craft butcher would know it, but comes as a 'protein booster' or 'broth'. Lentils aren't lentils but 'high viscosity pulse flour'. Cheese isn't cheese, but a 'goat flavour cheese powder'. Onions aren't onions but 'caramelised onion juice concentrate'.

If your company doesn't keep up with technical developments in the field, you can be sure that your competitors will, and the current drive to clean up labels puts manufacturers under further pressure to source new ingredients that do the job, but which sound better on the label. There's just so much to know. As the Danish R2 Group put it: 'Purchasing the right ingredient is no longer enough, and R2 Group therefore offers you all the **building blocks** [note the emphasis in bold] you need when innovating and producing food products.'

Once embarked on the modern processed food experiment, a manufacturer faces all manner of technical challenges never encountered by any home cook, and these require state-of-the-art ingredient know-how. For instance, at various stages in large-scale food processing, manufacturers can struggle with the problem of excessive foam. The answer to that issue is a product such as Silfoam®, a silicone-based system solution that controls 'foam-intensive applications' and 'facilitates smooth running processes'. This silicone product is also used in other industries, including 'textiles, detergents, cleaning products, pulp, petrochemicals, dispersions, pharmaceuticals, agrochemicals, food, biotech, fermentation or wastewater treatment sectors'.

Manufacturers who need their tomato sauce to be thick enough not to leak out of its plastic carton, smooth, and just a little bit glossy, so that it doesn't look matt and old after several days in the fridge, can see the advantages of Microlys®, a 'cost-effective' speciality starch that gives a product a 'shiny, smooth surface and high viscosity', or Pulpiz™, Tate & Lyle's tomato 'pulp extender'. Based on modified starch, its makers say that it gives the same pulpy visual appeal as an all-tomato sauce, using 25% less tomato paste. Companies that put added colour in their products may find that they stick to their equipment, forming clumps through the product, or 'migrating' from one part to another, from a sponge to an icing, say. These issues can be resolved by using colours in 'oil-dispersible technology' that guarantees a uniform effect every time.

If your company makes low-grade processed sausages, surimi, scampi or 'structured' (reformed) or 'injected' cooked hams with lots of added water, you'll probably be interested in using a product such as BDF's Probind®, made from an enzyme, transglutaminase, that will firm the meat up a bit and encourage liquid retention. As this enzyme is classified as a processing aid by the European Commission, you won't have to declare it on the label. Or perhaps you'd prefer to use a phosphate-based product, produced from phosphoric acid, such as Carfosel®, because it 'reduces thaw drip' and ensures 'a homogenous product'.

'Off flavours', which can come both from the extreme heat of the manufacturing process itself, the addition of additives, packaging, cleaning chemicals, rogue bacteria and many other sources, are another constant bugbear for large-scale food processors. But these can be 'masked' in many product formulations by adding a product such as 'dairy essence', which are concentrated cream and milk flavours 'unlocked' using enzyme technology, or simply by adding an assertive dose of flavouring, either 'natural' or synthetic.

A further occupational hazard of being a food manufacturer is that you have retailers leaning on you to reduce levels of ingredients in your products that are on the public health establishment's hit list. Salt is a case in point: the processed food industry has depended on it heavily to compensate for the depletion of natural flavour that comes hand-in-hand with industrial-scale food processing. Supermarkets like to sell processed food plastered with reassuring low-salt declarations and green traffic lights. Unfortunately for manufacturers, the obvious substitute is potassium chloride, but it has a bitter, metallic flavour. So manufacturers might well be tempted to try out Scelta Mushrooms®, a 'umami salt reduction tool', one of the latest industry answers to this pressing problem.

Food Ingredients 2013 was a veritable treasure trove of hugely clever food manufacturing ingredients such as these, but to the lay person, and, I suspect, many manufacturers, lots of them are a puzzle. Natural foods aren't shrouded in mystery. Meat, fish, dairy, fruit and vegetables – their production processes are well documented. But without an advanced grasp of chemistry and biology, it isn't possible to figure out what, precisely, most of these food manufacturing ingredients actually are, and how exactly they are produced.

Certainly the ingredient companies, although happy to make big claims for their products, are extremely reticent when asked to explain how they are made. Doing the rounds at Food Ingredients, I got into conversation with several company representatives keen to persuade me of the fantastic properties of their ingredients. But when I began to ask questions about how they were formulated, and what they contained, a definite reticence crept in, and my respondents began to answer like Ministry of Defence press officers. The best they could come up with were vague references to 'thermal' or 'mechanical' or 'enzymatic' treatments, or 'edible coating technology'. The parsimonious details of formulations offered, descriptions such as 'lactic acids with other ingredients', or 'contains natural nucleotides', or 'part of a revolutionary new generation of texturisers', left me little the wiser. Indeed, it was obvious that merely to seek a more informative answer instantly marked me out as an industry outsider, someone disinclined to accept claims for revolutionary new products uncritically without supporting documentation.

I was particularly drawn to the stand of Dohler, 'a global producer, marketer and provider of technology-based solutions to the food and beverage industry', by its vivid 'red brilliance' colouring 'from a 100 per cent natural source'. The basis of this colouring, I learned, is black carrot, grown mainly in Turkey, where the company's processing takes place. But how is this colour concentrate actually made, I asked? What does the processing involve? What needs to happen to a pile of carrots, harvested in a Turkish field, to transform it into a powerful, gleaming substance that can bestow on food and drink 'a fantastic colour spectrum ranging from warm and bright red hues to shining ruby tones all the way to blue shades of red'? The company's representatives obviously did not expect to answer such a query. 'It's a special process' was the only answer I could get.

Food Ingredients 2013 was full of products that are made by 'special' and 'unique' processes, 'innovative technologies' and 'sophisticated manufacturing methods', but the detail of them is never spelt out. No surprise there. The majority of the products that were on offer are protected by a little ® or ™ registered trademark symbol, which marks out a company's exclusive ownership of a product. The presence of the trademark signifies its intellectual property rights over a product and enables it to legally prevent others from copying or 'free riding' on its investment. From a consumer point of view, the trademark symbol also has another very important function: it allows companies to hide behind an ethos of commercial confidentiality and trade secrets to duck any less than superficial questions about how their products are actually made.

The brand names of many products being promoted at Food Ingredients did offer small clues as to their purpose.

Hydro-Fi™ is a 'high performance synergy of citrus fibre and hydrocolloids (essentially glues), designed to 'improve the yield of meatballs'. It is one of the latest products that use 'gum technology'. SuperStab™ (the sales material shows a glass of water with an oil-like substance swirling through it) is 'the ultimate natural emulsifier' made from 'an innovative proprietary process with specific raw material screening and preparation'. A yeast extract, Bionis®, boosts the 'meaty, condiment and umami flavour notes in frankfurters'. A 'speciality starch' called Culinar Keep promises 'prolonged shelf life of sensitive ingredients' so 'increasing productivity and savings costs'. Amongst other selling points, Meatshure®, an 'encapsulated acidulant', 'prevents protein extraction' and 'controls alginate reaction to yield desired binding'. The pitch for Cavamax®, various cyclodextrin formulations, is that they offer 'targeted protection and masking of specific flavourings'. Volactose is 'a whey permeate that 'allows exceptional handling in the manufacturing environment' producing 'superior surface browning'. A light brown liquid named Ecoprol, a melange of propyl gallate, citric acid, potassium sorbate, orthophosphoric acid, acetic acid and propylene glycol, sounded like a truly original fisherman's friend, because it 'extends the shelf life of fish, especially in the processing and marketing phase'.

Food manufacturing terminology is as linguistically taxing as a foreign language, and possibly even more impenetrable to the uninitiated, because the underlying concepts and semantics are so utterly different from those that underpin lay discussions of the properties of food.

Tired after hours of walking round Food Ingredients, and uncharacteristically, not feeling hungry, I sought refuge at a stand displaying cut up fruits and vegetables; it just felt so good to see something natural, something instantly recognisable as food in a sea of products that were quite the opposite. But why, I wondered, did they have dates, several weeks past, beside them? It was only in conversation with a salesman for Agricoat that I learned that the fruits had been dipped in one of its solutions, NatureSeal, which because it contains citric acid along with other unnamed ingredients, adds 21 days to their shelf life. Treated in this way, carrots don't develop that tell-tale white that makes them look old, cut apples don't turn brown, pears don't become translucent, melons don't ooze, and kiwis don't collapse into a jellied mush. As for leafy salads, a dip in NatureSeal leaves them 'appearing fresh and natural'.

For the salesman, this preparation was a technical triumph, a boon to caterers who would otherwise waste unsold food. And there was a further benefit. Because NatureSeal is classed as a processing aid, and not an ingredient, there is no need to declare it on the label, no obligation to tell consumers that their 'fresh' fruit salad was weeks old.

Somehow, I couldn't share his enthusiasm for NatureSeal's waste reduction potential because a disturbing thought had dropped into my mind. Had I eaten 'fresh' fruit salads treated in this way? Maybe I had bought a tub on a station platform, seeing it as the healthiest option in amongst an otherwise dire choice of junk? Or perhaps I had settled for it on a hotel buffet breakfast, thinking that it would be preferable to toast made from rubbish industrial bread?

And then a further penny dropped. Even though I was someone who never knowingly eats food with obscure ingredients that I don't recognise, I had probably consumed many of the wonder products at Food Ingredients 2013 unawares. So many of these products have been introduced, slowly and artfully, into ready-made, processed foods that many of us eat every day, in canteens, cafeterias, pubs, hotels, restaurants and takeaways that buy in and serve up factory-made products, everything from reheatable bistro meals and ready-to-bake baguettes, to ready-to-serve cheesecake and pre-rolled pizza bases. The fact is that we are all eating prepared foods made using such state-of-the-art food manufacturing technology, and mainly doing so unwittingly, either because these food components and aids don't need to be listed on the label, or because weasel words, such as 'flour' and 'protein', peppered with the liberal use of the adjective 'natural', do not give us the full flavour of their production method. What's more, we don't have a clue, and probably neither do many manufacturers, about what this novel diet might actually be doing to us.

Outside the exhibition halls, in the lobby, the movers and shakers of the food manufacturing world stood in huddles, cutting deals, swopping business cards and posing for photos for the next corporate brochure. Given the scarcity of anything truly food-like to graze on at Food Ingredients, it wasn't too surprising to see that a long queue had formed for a pop-up pretzel stand. I was almost tempted to join it until I found myself wondering whether, perhaps, those warm pretzels owed their humid chew, their sheen, their flavour, their colour, or their smell to some of the innovative products on display inside. Instead, with a spring in my step I headed for a breath of fresh air outdoors. Food Ingredients had seriously blunted my appetite, and only reconnecting with food in its natural state would kick it back into life.

5

Fresh in store

When you pop into an M&S food hall, you need a will of iron to walk past the in-store bakery without buying anything. After you have pushed your trolley down those sterile, odour-free, teeth-chatteringly cold aisles, past shelves banked high with convenience food in boxes, who isn't going to be seduced? The pleasing contours and golden hues of the assorted Viennoiserie, traybakes, muffins, tea breads, pastries and loaves create a visual architecture that primes us to expect real food in a fresh-from-the-oven state. That captivating aroma curls its way under the nose, stimulating the salivary glands, engendering feel-good thoughts of happy homes, nurturing childhoods and reassuring, dependable everyday pleasures. With its base notes of yeasty bread, buttery croissants and crusty scones, and its top notes of cinnamon, fragrant apple, vanilla and chocolate, you would make a fortune if you could distil and bottle this heart-melting scent: Parfum de Home Baking, the nation's comfort blanket.

Nowadays, many of the in-store bakeries at M&S are state-of-the-art. This is relatively recent. By the chain's own admission, they used to be behind the market in terms of sales and volume and were viewed as 'clinical, uninspiring, out of touch and with below-average food-hall profitability'. They looked utilitarian, just like the standard supermarket in-store bakery where any come-hither scents created must compete with the brash odours of the washing powder aisle, but then they were revamped. Now they are smartly kitted out with gleaming white-tiled walls, stylish pendant lights, and a floor that looks like timeless limestone. Everything on sale is displayed unwrapped in rustic wicker trays, in baskets resting on wooden crates, or on jute sacks; this creates a more informal homespun look and encourages you to help yourself. Staff wear chefs' whites under a linen-like apron, and a smart Nehru-style black cap, a mood board design ethos that combines the sophistication of Dean & DeLuca-style Manhattan deli chic with country barn.

The point of all this effort is to 'create theatre' in the food hall, 'drive purchase' of other items (that is, get customers to buy more of everything else), and help establish M&S's 'food credentials' as a specialist food retailer. This strategy has paid off handsomely. Profitability has tripled as the bakeries have seen record-breaking like-for-like growth.

These bakeries look and smell so good, you might just think 'Why on earth would I bother to bake?' Even for dedicated home bakers who sit glued to the latest round of *The Great British Bake Off* for nights on end, it is terribly tempting to hang up your pinny and just graze from the in-store bakery. After all, M&S is widely held to be a cut above the other chains, and those loaves, cakes, buns and muffins do look like something an Earth-goddess-mum-come-craft-baker would knock up – and with all the associated simple virtues. Strategically situated near the shelves of pre-wrapped bakery goods, these goodies seem, by comparison, positively homely and low-tech. But are they?

While all baked goods not made in an in-store bakery must, by law, come labelled with a complete list of every ingredient and additive in the mix, so that if you are interested, you can see what you will be eating, the same requirement does not apply to anything sold from in-store bakeries. Still, you'd think that progressive retailers would offer such information voluntarily.

I tried to find the ingredient listings for M&S in-store bakery products online. In the 'About our food' sections of the M&S website it simply said 'As some of our foods are freshly prepared in our stores, this page can help you find out the nutritional content'. It gave a breakdown for everything from the walnut loaf to the pecan and almond Danish pastry – how much fat, protein, salt, calories and so on – in one of those supposedly illuminating charts that purport to be the ultimate exercise in transparency, but which are more or less incomprehensible to anyone who isn't a professional dietician. Fulsome nutritional details, but no sign of an ingredient listing.

I then asked the M&S press centre to provide me with the information, and got back a civil, but unilluminating response:

> I'm afraid as we don't sell food online (other than our food to order), we don't have a central database that I can direct you to, so it's a bit tricky. If you could let me know the specific bakery products you'd like the ingredients for, I can certainly try to find out for you.

And was it just me, or was there a rising note of defensiveness in the final line:

> Would you also mind giving me a bit more info about the book – what's the angle you're looking at?

It sounded as though it could be like pulling teeth to extract ingredients lists via the regular press channels, so on a quiet Monday morning, I decided to visit an M&S in-store bakery in person, as a member of the public, thinking that this would be a more direct way to get an answer. I asked one of the women who was working away behind the baskets of bread and buns if I could see the ingredients listing for the products on sale. She looked a bit perplexed; this was clearly not a question she had been trained to answer. Still, trying to be helpful, she showed me information about allergens (soya, eggs, peanuts, etc.) and yet again, offered up that already familiar nutritional information. But, she said, there wasn't a list of ingredients as such, only a behind-the-counter product guide for the bakery staff's guidance. It did list ingredients by product, but she wasn't sure if she could let me see it. Why was I asking anyway? Knowing what's in your food should be a matter of public record, and the relevant information readily available, but it was beginning to feel like an off-the-wall, Freedom of Information Act request. Eventually, though, I managed to see a copy of the manual.

Flicking though the manual, it soon became apparent that there are quite a few nuggets of information contained within it that would act as a reality check for anyone who thinks that what they buy here isn't that different from the homemade equivalent. For starters, it knocks on the head the wishful thinking inherent in the term 'in-store bakery': the cosy notion that these products are created from scratch on the premises. The manual makes it clear that, on the contrary, the products are purchased, usually frozen and ready to be finished off in ovens, from named third-party bakery companies all over the UK, then sold as fresh. Several of these suppliers are well-known brands in the world of catering, supplying products to everything from train station takeaways and hotels to coffee shops and supermarket chains. This is why the products in those country fair baskets look hauntingly familiar. You will have seen them, or products very similar to them, on many occasions, and in various settings.

First up was the M&S jam doughnut. The functional product description in the manual is as follows: 'A doughnut, deep fried in vegetable oil and injected with raspberry jam filling. Supplied with four plastic bags per case. Using these bags, doughnuts to be coated with approximately three grams of sugar in-store.' The product sheet makes clear that the doughnuts arrive cooked and frozen and can be kept that way for nine months. All that the 'bakers' had to do was put them through the oven on a set programme (number 7 in the case of doughnuts, which is 120°C for eight minutes, followed by 100°C for three minutes), then allow them to cool before sugaring them in the bags provided. Et les voilà, nice 'fresh' doughnuts!

The same push-button method of baking applied to other items on sale. Once these products are delivered to the store – either unbaked or part-baked, and frozen – staff simply had to bake them off at a specified oven programme: French apple pastries (Programme 15), custard pastries (Programme 17), cinnamon croissants (Programme 5), bread rolls (Programme

12), and so on. Perhaps the Real Bread Campaign was overstating its point when it described such in-store bakeries as 'tanning salons' for products that have been made in industrial bakery plants elsewhere, and joked about the 'Great British Fake-Off', but you can see what it was getting at.

Baking method apart, the product information sheet did indeed provide a comprehensive ingredient listing, which covered some items you'd expect to find (flour, yeast, oil, sugar) and others that you might not (wheat gluten, ascorbic acid, dextrose, soya flour). While a homemade raspberry jam contains only two items – raspberries and sugar – this 'raspberry jam filling' was an amalgam of sugar syrup, raspberry purée, pectin, citric acid and calcium chloride E509, a 'sequestrant' chemical that acts as a preservative and firming agent. So the red stuff in your M&S doughnut was raspberry jam of sorts, but not jam as the Women's Institute would know it.

The Bakewell tart, supplied frozen and unbaked, with a freezer life of six months, offered another spin on raspberry jam, with ingredients that echo the jam filling in the doughnut, only this time it also included two different sugar syrups, sucrose syrup and glucose-fructose syrup, the latter a relatively modern formulation that health campaigners in the USA believe is helping to drive the obesity epidemic.

And it was the same story with everything else on sale here – they all contained ingredients you won't find in any home baker's larder or, for that matter, in the kitchen of any self-respecting pastry chef. The ingredients in a homemade classic crème pâtissière would be milk, egg yolks, sugar, cornflour and a vanilla pod, or vanilla extract. But the crème pâtissière in the pain aux raisins, yet again supplied pre-prepared and frozen, was made from water, sugar, modified potato starch, dry whey (a milk protein), dried milk, maltodextrin (a starch that helps increase volume to create what food manufacturers refer to as 'a rich mouthfeel'), xanthan gum (a gluey thickener), a product charmingly called 'spent vanilla seeds', as well as flavouring and colouring.

Similarly, the first ingredient in the chocolate-filled muffins was not flour, but sugar; its further ingredients include glycerine, modified maize starch, three different E-numbered emulsifiers, dried whey, dried protein, guar gum (used as a 'stabiliser') and flavouring.

A toothsome Danish pastry contained pectin (to provide a smooth, elastic gel structure in the custard), isomalt (a sugar alcohol), whey protein, flavouring, a gelling agent, an acidity regulator, a preservative, and mixed carotenes for colouring. The latter additive is derived either from plants or algae obtained by fermentation of a fungus, *Blakeslea trispora*. Put it this way, it's not the sort of kit that your average home baker has to hand.

As I photographed the product sheets, the enticing scent of the still warm cinnamon twists was making me feel ravenous, but then I saw its ingredients, which included potato starch, sodium alginate, xanthan gum, and agar (thickeners), enzyme (exact nature and purpose unspecified), calcium carbonate (a type of chalk), and colour, and it suddenly lost its winsome appeal.

Bear in mind though that in 'baking off' pre-made frozen breads and pastries, M&S is only doing what all the other supermarket chains do, and because our big grocery chains often use the same third party, industrial bakery product companies, it seems not unreasonable to assume that the ingredients used, while they might vary a little, will not be hugely dissimilar.

Would takeaways be any different, I wondered? So it was off – where else? – to Greggs, Britain's oldest and largest bakery chain. With more bakery shops than McDonald's has burger bars, it is beginning to look every bit as much of a national institution as M&S. 'We're proud to be keeping the craft of fresh baking alive', says Greggs. 'Our bakers bake daily to our own unique recipes.' Furthermore, Greggs boasts that 'all the food we make is free from artificial colours, hydrogenated fats, and has no trans fats', which sounds promising. The bragging doesn't stop there:

> We're proud to keep the art of the confectioner alive in our bakeries. We insist on using quality ingredients, like the tangy flavouring from Sicilian lemons and rich Belgian chocolate in our gorgeous muffins. Our dedicated confectioners always strive for perfection, many of our sweet treats are finished by hand. Our Yum Yums are hand-twisted and the cream on our cream cakes is piped by hand in true craft bakery style.

Mmm, hand-twisted Yum Yums, now that certainly gets the gastric juices flowing.

Because Greggs so clearly takes such a craft pride in its bakery art, surely it would be keen to provide me with further chapter and verse? Once again, its ingredients list seemed the obvious place to start. Walking into one of its town centre shops, which seems to be steadily busy from breakfast through lunch until tea-time, I posed the same question as I had at M&S – where is the ingredient list? – and got the same response. A pleasant woman behind the counter gave me a copy of a customer information leaflet headed 'From wheat to eat', with an expansive-looking section headed 'What goes into your favourite savouries', but yet again – groundhog day – in amongst the marketing spin, the only hard facts offered were a product-by-product nutritional breakdown: calories, energy value and so on. I reiterated that I was looking for ingredients listings. She shot me a your-guess-is-as-good-as-mine look, then pointed to the wall, where unobtrusive next to the chiller cabinets filled with sandwiches and soft drinks, was a terse customer advice notice. This still didn't give me the full disclosure I was looking for, but it did offer a few hard facts, required by law, such as:

> Products sold on these premises contain one or more of the following – additives, antioxidants, sweeteners, colours, flavourings, flavour enhancers, preservatives.

More informative in a specific sort of way was the 'typical meat contents' information for savoury products, often described as 'man snacks' because of their supposedly sustaining carnivorous contents. This showed, for example, that the pork element in a Greggs jumbo sausage roll accounted for just 19 per cent of the total ingredients – not much in the way of primal food – and that the pork contained natural colour and preservative.

It was a similar story with the chicken bake: the chicken element accounted for only 18 per cent of the ingredients, and the chicken itself contained natural flavour and natural colour. Bridies, Scotch pies, steak bakes, fajita chicken lattices and more, all contained a colour, flavour or preservative, and some contained all three. And there were a few more intriguing flashes of detail. It stated, for instance, that 'ham used in some of our products is formed from selected cuts of pure pork leg', which is to say that it wasn't cut from a whole ham in the traditional sense of that word. It also informed me that the 'breakfast sausage contains beef protein', but it didn't tell me what, exactly, 'beef protein' is, as opposed to straight beef as we know it. After all, beef is naturally rich in protein, so why the semantic word play? Had beef protein in some other form been added to pork sausage? This wording didn't enlighten me.

Nevertheless, the customer notice was rounded off with an upbeat and generous flourish: 'If you have any queries, do not hesitate to ask the staff in the shop who will be pleased to help you'. Well, I had tried that, but they didn't seem to know the full story either. So I contacted the public relations company that handles media enquiries for Greggs, and asked for the ingredients listings for their products. 'We'll look into this for you', they promised. In a week, I hadn't heard a thing, so I followed up my request. Three weeks later, I received this response from the senior manager handling the Greggs account:

> Unfortunately whilst nutritional information is available on the Greggs website, ingredient lists are not because Greggs wishes to protect the recipes of its iconic products.

In other words, get lost. We don't need, by law, to tell you what's in our products, so we're not going to. Greggs just wanted me to take it on trust that it puts only the freshest and finest ingredients into its 'iconic products'. And yet, in the absence of reassuring transparency, I felt unable to do so.

PART TWO

The defining characteristics of processed food

6

Sweet

Jason Reitman's black comedy about the dark art of lobbying, *Thank You for Smoking*, starred Aaron Eckhart as a high-earning lobbyist for the tobacco industry. At one point in the film, Eckhart is seen in cynical conversation with fellow professional lobbyists (for the alcohol industry and gun lobby) debating who amongst them has the toughest reason and evidence-denying job. Were he making that film now, Reitman might well put a lobbyist for the sugar industry around the table, because sugar is in big trouble, and needs all the help it can get. Despite their best efforts, sugar companies and sugar-dependent manufacturers find themselves in a deep, defensive silo, as sticky, dark and hard to get out of as treacle. Sugar, as the headlines read, is the new tobacco.

Changed days. When saturated fat was the nutrition establishment's wicker man, the health-wrecking effects of sugar sneaked in under the radar. The fatwa on fat was a cash cow for sugar refiners, spawning legions of processed products with ramped-up levels of sugar to cover up the inevitable loss of taste that occurs when flavour-centric fat is removed.

So fixated was the dietetic establishment with promoting fat avoidance, that, on occasion, it even ended up promoting sugar because the healthiness of foods was defined by the absence of fat. In 2014 a baffled friend of mine was given a copy of a document known as the Good Hearted Glasgow Diet Sheet by her GP on the grounds that she had high cholesterol. The introduction read: 'Cutting down on the amount of fat which you eat will help lower the level of cholesterol in your blood.' This is a highly debatable statement because the putative link between fat consumption and raised cholesterol is based on over-simplistic science, as is the contention that reducing cholesterol improves health outcomes. The vexed question of cholesterol apart, it was alarming to read the diet advice: sugar, jam, marmalade, honey, boiled sweets, pastilles and gums all appeared in the 'recommended foods' column.

Simmering away in the background, of course, there has long been a persistent narrative on sugar and its capacity to damage our health. Back in 1972, physiologist John Yudkin published his book, *Sweet and Dangerous*, subsequently retitled more explicitly in further editions as *Pure, White, and Deadly: How Sugar Is Killing Us and What We Can Do to Stop It*. If that message isn't clear enough, what is? But for many years, the sugar lobby suppressed such explicit attack, using a two-pronged strategy.

The first tactic was to neutralise any embedded concerns about sugar we might have by creating a spurious positive association with health. The aim here is to create a feel-good message that clashes with, and hopefully overrides, any negative perception. (This is a classic damage-limitation manoeuvre used by potentially unpopular companies, the reason why polluting oil companies often sponsor wildlife projects, for example.)

In the case of companies whose products are loaded with sugar, the easiest response was to link their products to sport, athleticism and physical activity. So Coca-Cola was all too happy to be the official soft drinks provider for the London 2012 Olympic Games as this enabled it to demonstrate its strong commitment to the 'Olympic values – participation, friendship, excellence and respect', and 'build deeper relationships with the people who enjoy our products'. Isn't that nice? Irn-Bru, the amber-coloured, sweet fizzy drink 'made in Scotland from girders' by A.G. Barr, was declared the 'Official Soft Drink of Glasgow' for the 2014 Commonwealth Games. Bear in mind that Glasgow is the city with the lowest life expectancy in the UK, in the country (Scotland) that has the worst health record in Europe. 'Retailers will be able to generate excellent visibility in-store with the point of sale [material] we are providing and capitalise on the unrivalled opportunity to drive soft drinks' sales before, during and after Glasgow 2014', the company's head of marketing purred. However much purveyors of sweet products appear to encourage physical exercise, it's clear that upping sales is their overriding preoccupation.

The sugar lobby's second tactic was not on show in any public sports arena, but highly effective behind the scenes: it dismissed its critics as mavericks and heretics on the fringes of scientific consensus. In the case of John Yudkin, who first blew the whistle on sugar, his stance cost him dearly. Jobs and research grants that might otherwise have come Yudkin's way did not materialise, and attacks on him included the abrupt cancellation of conferences where he might advance the anti-sugar case. The sugar lobby dismissed *Pure, White, and Deadly* as a work of fiction, and continued for decades to bullishly pursue anyone who dared to disseminate any anti-sugar views.

I have first-hand experience of this. In 2009, a representative of the UK sugar lobby, then known as the Sugar Bureau, a body that has since changed its name to the less partisan and more scientific-sounding Sugar Nutrition UK, wrote to my editor at a popular magazine, demanding that I provide scientific evidence to justify every reference I had made about the negative impact of sugar on health in an article. He even asked, without any hint of irony, that I back up my assertion that sugar can cause tooth decay, a statement that had been uncontroversial for decades. Nevertheless, all this I duly did, at some length, and in time-consuming detail.

Not satisfied with my response, the pugnacious sugar lobby representative referred the matter back to my editor. She batted the complaint upstairs to the department that deals with legal affairs. It was already well acquainted with sugar lobby complaints as a result of its habit of stamping on any journalist, editor or broadcaster who dared to let it be said that sugar might be anything other than good for us. In my case, the sugar lobby eventually gave up, but for years this general strategy paid off. It effectively silenced critics by keeping them tied up in lengthy, work-intensive exchanges of letters, constantly refusing to accept their very credible sources and demanding that letters 'correcting' the 'misleading' and outlandish notion that sugar isn't good for you, be printed. Knowing how combative and demanding the sugar lobby was, editors and journalists tended to self-censor, by avoiding the subject, or writing about it in a softly-softly, inoffensive way. To do otherwise would probably mean getting caught up in a protracted, seemingly interminable dialogue.

The media soon got the message: 'Don't say anything negative about sugar unless you're up for a lorry load of hassle.'

Try as hard as they might, lobbyists can only suppress bad news for so long. In the words of one *British Medical Journal* editorial, 'the pendulum is now definitely swinging away from fat as the root of all evil'. As the nutritional case against saturated fat has begun melting away, sugar has replaced it as public health enemy number one. The global sugar lobby really began to feel the heat in 2012 with the publication of Dr Robert Lustig's book, *Fat Chance*, which powerfully argued that sugar, not fat, is the real villain in the global obesity epidemic. Publication in the science journal *Nature* of an article written by Dr Lustig and two colleagues, entitled 'The Toxic Truth About Sugar', upped the temperature further. It argued persuasively that an excess of sugar contributes to 35 million deaths a year worldwide, by making us fat, disrupting our metabolism, raising blood pressure, throwing hormones off balance and damaging the liver.

By 2014, the case against sugar was bubbling up uncontrollably all over the place, like an untended saucepan of rapidly darkening, blisteringly hot caramel. And when the World Health Organization announced draft guidance recommending that people should halve their maximum daily intake of free sugars – that's added sugars, including those from honey, syrups and fruit juice – from 10 per cent of total calories to 5 per cent, citing growing concern about sugar's contribution to obesity and dental diseases, sugar was obviously on the back foot.

True to type, companies up to their necks in sugar continued to mount the same old defence. Major refiner, AB Sugar, complained loudly that sugar was being singled out unfairly as the leading culprit in the obesity epidemic. Buying time, CAOBISCO, the Association of Chocolate, Biscuits and Confectionery Industries of Europe, tried to muddy the waters by insisting that the scientific case against sugar required 'further scientific substantiation'. The British Nutrition Foundation, which, despite its neutral, professorial name, is a partisan defender of industrial food production, hailed the 'sugar is the new tobacco' attack as 'misleading', clinging to its dog-eared script that sugar is only harmful in excess, and nutritionally necessary otherwise. 'Sugar', it says, 'is a type of carbohydrate that provides energy for the body in the form of glucose. In particular the brain needs glucose to function, as do muscles during exercise'. Far from sugar being bad for us, we are asked to believe that sugar is actually necessary for our bodies to function properly. Using this logic, candy floss can be a desirable part of a 'balanced' diet.

Disturbingly, the founder of one baby food company wrote passionately that 'outrageous headlines' were 'simplifying this serious national issue to a single, too simple, witch-hunt of one foodstuff'. What infant needs sugar added to its food? And when I wrote a column for the *Grocer* magazine saying that we had to face facts and cut our consumption of sugar, Terry Jones, the director of the Food and Drink Federation – a body that acts as a mouthpiece for the processed food and drink industry – responded with yet another letter to the editor:

> Although the balance of scientific evidence shows that sugars, like any other nutrient, can be enjoyed as part of a varied and balanced diet, a vocal minority persist in demonising this ingredient. The simple balanced diet and physical activity message has lost out to alarming narratives.

That exasperated final line expressed a dawning realisation in the food industry that sugar has been outed as public health enemy Number One, and there is no going back. The defence of sugar is doomed. However much the sugar lobby blusters, it has lost its war, leaving manufacturers vulnerable to criticism for using it in such great quantity, and under immense pressure to reduce added sugar content in food and beverages. These days, mention of sugar on a product is not quite as bad as having a skull and crossbones on the label, but it is heading that way.

From a public relations and sales point of view, that troublesome, toxic word 'sugar' has to be shooed off labels as fast as possible, and supermarkets have to be seen to be responding. Waitrose, for example, announced in 2014 that it was adjusting and reformulating its chilled juice and smoothie range, removing 7.1 tonnes of sugar a year, a gesture of commitment towards the new reduced sugar era. This meant delisting several lines in PepsiCo's Copella and Tropicana range. Product delistings such as these send shock waves through the processed food industry. Ouch, that hurts! What's next for the chop?

Yet even under heavy pressure from supermarkets, there's only so much sugar manufacturers can shed because they rely so heavily on a sweet taste to construct their products. A 100 gram, one-person can of cola contains up to nine teaspoons of sugar and, if you think about it, many highly profitable soft drinks are essentially water with sugars or sweeteners, colours and flavourings added – and this includes many products sold as juices, not just soft drinks.

Sugar is not only a cornerstone of manufactured drinks, confectionery, bakery, breakfast cereals and desserts, but also a surprisingly important ingredient in many savoury products: mayonnaise, ketchup, soups and pasta sauces, ready meals, gravy and bread. When *Which?* investigated ready meals, it found that Sainsbury's sweet and sour chicken with rice, and Tesco's Everyday Value sweet and sour chicken with rice, contained around ten teaspoons of sugar in a meal for one. Sweetness is a hallmark of the lion's share of processed foods.

Sugar also has lots of other important technological properties for food manufacturers. It makes drinks more viscous and acts as a preservative in foods with long best before dates. Its water-binding property helps moisture retention, so you feel like you're getting more for your money. Knowing we eat with our eyes, manufacturers use it to create enticing golden crusts and the appearance of patiently roasted meat. Added sugar makes dough more voluminous. In the words of one industry report, 'sugar provides bulk, textural elements, browning, caramelisation and other necessary functional elements [in food manufacture] beyond its sweet taste'. In fact, telling food manufacturers to go easy on the sugar is like asking a builder to construct a house without joists.

Sugar is such a lynchpin of food and drink manufacture, reformulating products so that they contain less, or none, is far from straightforward: it cannot usually be replaced by a single ingredient. Removing or replacing sugar will change taste, texture and appearance. To compensate, the whole recipe needs to be reformulated. So the hunt is on to find an alternative sweet substance with all the functional attributes needed in large-scale food and drink processing, one that can plausibly be presented to the public as more benign than sugar.

Now, the food industry has been quietly working on losing mentions of the toxic word 'sugar' on its products for quite some time, using a series of ploys. Foremost here was the grooming of fructose, the type of sugar found naturally in fruit, for its role as a healthier type of sugar. This worked for a while. As every junk food marketer knows, the mere mention of fruit is a shortcut to creating a healthy image for a product. Fruit sugar sounds so much more health-enhancing than plain old sugar, doesn't it? However, while the fructose in whole fruit comes hand-in-hand with fibre, which slows and reduces the body's absorption of sugar, this is not the case when fructose is added in a highly refined, 100 per cent purified form, as it is in processed foods. When Mother Nature designed fruit, she thought it through properly. The potential poison in it (fructose) comes in the same wrapper as the antidote (fibre), which seems to prevent the former having any negative effects on our metabolism. But when pure fructose is used in food manufacture, it is every bit as disastrous for health as sucrose, the more familiar white table sugar; some scientists argue that its effect is even worse. Indeed, fructose now looks like the once promising new pupil in the class who turned out to be a nightmare.

Of intense concern has been the highly refined form of fructose, extracted from corn using enzyme technology, called high fructose corn syrup (HFCS). In the UK, it more commonly appears on labels as glucose/fructose syrup, or vice versa. It is widely used in food manufacturing because it is cheaper than sugar and being liquid, it is easier to handle in industrial-scale production. Consumption of this sweetener has been linked to gout, hypertension, fatty liver disease, type 2 diabetes and obesity. North American corn refiners continue to argue that HFCS is 'safe, natural and nutritionally the same as sugar', but it has become so hot to handle that consumers on both sides of the Atlantic are voting with their feet and avoiding it. David Rosenthal, Senior Vice-President of the US Corn Refiners Association, voiced the industry's image problem:

> This [bad] publicity has led to a subsequent set of misperceptions among some food and beverage marketers and manufacturers that a large number of consumers are actively avoiding brands with HFCS – and that switching to sugar in their formulations (and touting 'HFCS-free' on their labels) can improve their sales.

Stuck with a product that had garnered such an unenviable reputation, corn refiners came up with the idea of reinventing HFCS. Why not rename it as 'corn sugar'? Even the tainted word sugar didn't have such negative connotations as HFCS. Nice try, but this initiative was a sign of desperation, and even with the lobbying power of corn refiners, doomed to failure: the US Food and Drug Administration rejected the name change, so HFCS is still saddled with its image problem.

Cane sugar companies, meanwhile, have attempted a similar rebranding exercise with sugar, by trying to rename dried cane syrup, which is essentially an ever so slightly less refined type of sugar comparable to 'golden' cane sugar, as 'evaporated cane juice'. In 2009, the Food and Drug Administration also refused to authorise this term, on the grounds that it 'falsely suggests the sweeteners are juice'. Juice, courtesy of its association with fruit, shines that ever welcome 'wellness' glow on a product. Since 2012, US courts have seen several class action lawsuits against prominent companies on the grounds that evaporated cane juice is nothing more than sugar, cleverly disguised. One such case, against leading yogurt manufacturer Chobani, was dismissed, but others are following in its footsteps. Although the agency has repeatedly told food manufacturers not to use the term because it is false and misleading, it says that it has not reached a final decision, so companies determined to swop the word 'sugar' for 'juice' are still in with a fighting chance.

Seeing all the shenanigans around sugar and high fructose corn syrup, you might think that manufacturers could fall back on the option of high-intensity artificial sweeteners – after all, there is quite a collection of them. They include Aspartame, Acesulfame K, saccharin and Sucralose, which are respectively 200, 200, 300 and 600 hundred times sweeter than sucrose, the standard white refined sugar, but they are zero calorie. These chemically synthesised sweeteners have been around for decades and are widely used in diet drinks and foods, chewing gum and table-top sweeteners. Or a manufacturer could play around with the toothsome possibilities presented by the more recently developed neotame, which is a dizzying 8,000–13,000 times sweeter than sucrose. If that won't do the trick, a further high-intensity sweetener to consider is advantame. Made from aspartame and vanillin, it is an unimaginable 37,000 times sweeter than sugar. The European Union's Panel on Food Additives decided in 2014 that advantame raised 'no genotoxicity [damage to our DNA] or carcinogenicity concerns' at the levels permitted in food and drink.

Looking forward to trying advantame? Perhaps not. Although arguably artificial sweeteners have a more favourable reputation than high fructose corn syrup, and come with all manner of official reassurance, they can't seem to shake off safety concerns. Studies have linked artificial sweetener consumption to a variety of negative health effects: migraine, epilepsy, premature birth and brain cancer. Nevertheless, the European Food Safety Authority has ruled that all the sweeteners it permits for sale in the European Union, although potentially toxic in larger quantities, are 'safe for human consumption at current levels of exposure'. This may be reassuring to those who trust our regulators to put public health before corporate interests, but lingering health concerns around artificial sweeteners persist; several feature on Whole Foods Market's 'black list' of unacceptable ingredients, alongside HFCS. For manufacturers keen to dump sugar and HFCS for something that plays better with a critical public, embracing sweeteners may look like a case of out of the frying pan, into the fire.

From a more practical point of view, plain old sugar, or sucrose, has what's regarded in the food industry as the ideal bell curve flavour profile, that is, the taste starts off gently, builds to a pleasing peak, then fades away cleanly, whereas artificial sweeteners are often slow to build and have a lingering bitter, slightly metallic, almost liquorice-like aftertaste. That's not a problem in a product like chewing gum where the pungent mint will hide it, but it can stick out like a sore thumb elsewhere.

Safety and taste apart, a further blot on the horizon for artificial sweeteners is a growing body of evidence indicating that despite their absence of calories, they don't seem to do what they are meant to do, that is, help control weight. Indeed, several large-scale studies have found a positive correlation between artificial sweetener use and weight gain. One animal study found that rats consuming artificial sweetener gained weight faster than those eating the sugar. Some studies also flag up that artificial sweeteners could be worse for health than sugar. In 2013, a major study of over 66,000 women, tracking their consumption of sugar-sweetened and artificially-sweetened (diet) soft drinks over 14 years, found that those consuming the latter had a higher incidence of type 2 diabetes than those drinking the former. Later that year, a wide-ranging review of studies looking at the impact of artificial sweeteners on weight and other health outcomes reached this overall conclusion:

> Accumulating evidence suggests that frequent consumers of these sugar substitutes may also be at increased risk of excessive weight gain, metabolic syndrome, type 2 diabetes, and cardiovascular disease.

Surprised? After all, if artificial sweeteners contain no calories, how could they make you fat? One possibility is that a sweet taste, unaccompanied by the calories that come with conventional sugar, sends the body on a calorie hunt, seeking out those missing calories elsewhere, so encouraging over-eating. While classic sugar leaves us feeling content, it has been suggested that 'sweetness decoupled from caloric content offers partial, but not complete, activation of the food reward pathways'. In other words, artificial sweeteners awaken the brain's pleasure centre but don't deliver the anticipated satisfaction. So, for instance, although we choose the diet drink thinking that we are making a healthier choice, it could leave us craving a doughnut. Another theory is that artificial sweeteners wreak havoc with our appetite-regulating hormones, leptin and ghrelin, making us more liable to overeat.

Currently, what manufacturers crave is a 'no-sugar sugar', a dream-ticket substance that supplies the all-essential sweet taste, but one that has none of the health and safety baggage that attaches to sugar, HFCS and artificial sweeteners. Food and drink manufacturers know that consumers see 'natural' as good and 'processed' as bad, so if they want to have a healthy positioning in the market, the strategy is to go natural. Traditional sweeteners such as honey, maple syrup, coconut and palm sugar don't hit the spot for food manufacturers because they are much more expensive than sugar, HFCS and artificial sweeteners. They also taste too much of themselves, so they don't have the requisite neutrality to work in a wide range of products. Natural sweeteners, unless highly refined, exhibit a spectrum of flavours – treacle, caramel, smoky, resinous, butterscotch and so on – and this character gets in the way for food and drink manufacturers.

A few years back, agave syrup, sometimes sold with the more exotic title agave nectar, had a star billing in health food stores as a healthier substitute for sugar. It is derived from a spiky, cactus-like South American plant, and is about one and a half times sweeter than sugar. Here's how one agave brand promotes itself:

> The Aztecs prized the agave as a gift from the gods and used the liquid from its core to flavor foods and drinks. Now, due to increasing awareness of agave nectar's many beneficial properties, it is becoming the preferred sweetener of health conscious consumers, doctors, and natural foods cooks alike.

Agave nectar is often labelled as raw, but it is actually extracted either at a low temperature, or using enzymes. In its less processed form, dark agave syrup has a slight caramel flavour, but in its lighter, purer forms, it is mild and anonymous, characteristics that tick two key food-processing boxes. However, agave's image and commercial prospects took a nosedive when initial enthusiasm was tempered by a long, hard look at its chemical composition. Agave syrup has a higher fructose content than HFCS, and in the words of one food campaigner, 'most agave nectar or agave syrup is nothing more than a laboratory-generated super-condensed fructose syrup, devoid of virtually all nutrient value'.

As the agave moon has waned, another natural and traditional-sounding sweetener has twinkled brightly in the sugar-free firmament. Stevia, a leafy plant native to central and South America, where, we are told, it was traditionally chewed and used in teas by native populations, is the next great white hope for sugar redemption. Like agave, stevia has a covetable wisdom-of-the-ancients backstory that is a gift to marketing departments but, unlike agave, its trump card is that it is zero calorie.

Stevia is finding its way into soft drinks and manufactured food. In 2013, Coca-Cola started using Truvia®, the Cargill company's stevia-based sweetener, in Sprite, which allowed it to reduce the sugar content of this beverage by 30%. Coca-Cola stresses stevia's naturalness and ancient lineage: 'The stevia plant is a relative of the chrysanthemum, native to Paraguay, and has been used to sweeten drinks ever since indigenous people first discovered its flavour. It has been grown, harvested and used in South America for around 200 years.'

Don't you just love the sales pitch? But just how natural, exactly, is commercial stevia? It would seem that there is a world of difference between the sweet green stevia leaves chewed and brewed by native populations, and purified, highly concentrated chemicals extracted from these leaves. For starters, these modern stevia extracts are much sweeter. Whereas dried green leaves of stevia are a relatively feeble 40 times sweeter than sugar, the chemical extracts isolated from these leaves are 200–300 times sweeter. And while stevia leaves in their whole unprocessed state contain a raft of compounds – diterpene glycosides – that contribute to their sweetness, the stevia extracts that are already on the market, or in development, generally isolate only one or two glycosides from the plant. Truvia, Cargill's product 'born from the leaves of the stevia plant' uses one particular glycoside, rebaudioside A (reb A), and combines this with other ingredients. The major ingredient in Truvia is not stevia, but erythritol, a polyol, of which more below. Truvia also contains flavourings. 'Natural flavors are used to bring out the best of Truvia® natural sweetener, like pepper or salt or any other spice that would be used to enhance the taste of food', the company explains.

In the USA, Cargill has found itself defending class action lawsuits disputing Truvia's claim to naturalness. One such action complained that 'reb-A is not the natural crude preparation of stevia' so its manufacture is not 'similar to making tea', as Cargill's packaging suggests. Rather, it is 'a highly chemically processed and purified form of stevia-leaf extract'. The complaint also stated that the main ingredient in Truvia, erythritol, is 'synthetically made'. To date, such lawsuits have been settled out of court, with Cargill saying that they want to avoid the time and expense associated with further litigation. They have also agreed to modify their tagline in certain areas. Meanwhile, any manufacturer initially inclined to view stevia as a safe pair of hands might be having second thoughts.

And even if disputes over the use of the word 'natural' to describe highly processed stevia products could be resolved, there's still no getting away from stevia's less than perfect taste profile. One of the reasons stevia is only used to replace up to 30 per cent of the sugar in food and drink is its lingering, slightly cooling, almost mentholated aftertaste, reminiscent of liquorice or quinine. Sales of Sprite nosedived after stevia was added to the recipe. One influential panellist in an industry blind tasting suggested why: 'The aftertaste [of stevia] was strong and unpleasant.' Scientists are isolating more minor glycosides from stevia that might taste better. In theory, plant geneticists could breed the 'next' stevia: cultivars with higher levels of the more desirable glycosides. For the time being, although Stevia is the current sweetheart of the global high-intensity sweeteners market, it doesn't look like a prêt-à-porter solution for sugar reduction.

If stevia is still something of an unknown quantity for most people, what on earth are we to make of polyols, yet another emerging group of sweeteners? They appear on product labels by name – erythritol, mannitol, sorbitol, isomalt, lactitol, xylitol are the most common – and because European regulators regard them as additives, they each have an E number. But what exactly are they? Also called sugar alcohols, polyols are used as bulk sweeteners. Most are made in an industrial process by treating sugars – glucose, fructose, lactose, xylose – with hydrogen in the presence of a nickel catalyst. Polyols can also be produced by fermentation.

Erythritol, for instance, is produced from dextrose in corn, in a fermentation process that is catalysed by the introduction of a strain of yeast.

Some polyols, especially xylitol, absorb heat when dissolved in the mouth, causing a cooling effect – a property that's handy in chewing gums, but not that many other products, so this limits their usefulness to food processors. The main consumer selling point for polyols is that because they are only partially digested in the gut, they have a lower calorific value, but this putative benefit has a murky underbelly: they can also cause fermentation in the lower gut, producing diarrhoea and flatulence. This is why, in the EU, products that are more than 10 per cent composed of them must carry a warning label that 'excessive consumption can cause a laxative effect'. As a wholesale alternative to sugar, sugar alcohols are about as solid an option as mud.

All around the globe, scientists funded by big food and drink corporations are energetically questing after a problem-free sugar substitute that can be commercialised profitably and presented as natural. Much attention is being lavished on monk fruit, also known as Luo Han Guo, an Asian melon-like gourd, which contains compounds (mogrosides) that are 300 times sweeter than sugar. Just like stevia, in its raw, unprocessed, unsynthesised form, it has a venerable history of use, this time in Eastern traditional medicine. Monk fruit-derived sweeteners are hitting US shelves in cereals, drinks and meal replacers, but are not yet approved in the EU. Does this new contender have a rosy commercial future? The recent history of sugar substitutes has been one sorry serial tale of new generation miracle products that try – and fail – to fix the problems of the ones that went before. After the initial honeymoon period, flavour of the moment sweeteners have all foundered when informed consumers have caught up with how they are made. As one global trends analyst puts it:

> Natural sweeteners like those based on stevia and monk fruit, which are in vogue right now, may not have such an easy ride further down the line. The level of processing that these ingredients undergo is quite considerable, and consumers may, in time, turn against them in their quest for more natural options.

But what more natural option is there? Given the chequered history of sugar substitutes, one can't help wondering if finding an alternative to the gold standard taste and performance of sugar (sucrose) is a mission impossible, for nothing else seems to provide its unique flavour, nor fill the mouth in that pleasing way. Food engineers can use polyols to reproduce its mouthfeel and round out the brashness of artificial sweeteners. They can blend these with synthetic flavourings and acids in a vain attempt to disguise the slow build-up of sweet flavour, and cover up obtrusive aftertastes. In the words of one beverage scientist, 'an integration of polyols, nutritive [calorie containing] sweeteners, high intensity sweeteners and flavours allows our ingredient experts to achieve a more sucrose-like sweet perception'. But it's still not enough. All they can do is ape sugar; they can't match it.

And anyway, if it proves to be correct that a sweet taste, in and of itself, encourages us to want more of the same, then the hunt for sugar substitutes is a fool's errand. The literature of taste science shows a strong correlation between a person's customary intake of a flavour and his or her preferred intensity for that flavour. We know, for instance, that the more chilli you eat, the more you enjoy high levels of chilli in your food. If the cook puts one piquant green chilli in a curry, regular chilli eaters will find it too mild, while irregular chilli eaters will find it way too hot. Children accustomed to bland modern apple varieties, such as Gala, which have been bred to taste sweet, can find traditional varieties with their higher acidity levels too sharp. Taste isn't fixed but learned, based on culture, experience and familiarity. Judged against the muted sugar levels in Japanese confectionery, a cube of British fudge seems absurdly sugary and cloying. There is no universal baseline for sweetness the world over. Perception of sweetness is relative.

With sugar, as with everything else in life, we can't have our cake and eat it. However you try to dress up and repackage it, sugar is bad news, and candidates to replace it, no better. Addressing the very real possibility that we need to curb our desire for a sweet taste may prove to be an altogether more productive line of enquiry. If we want to be healthier, then the answer most likely lies in 'unsweetening' our diet: consuming less of any ingredient or additive that tastes sweet, irrespective of its source, production method, composition, or the calories it contains. Drinks are the first place to start, because it is so much easier to *drink* excessive amounts of sugar than it is to *eat* them. Drinking water rather than soft drinks and juice, and cutting down, then gradually eliminating sugar in tea and coffee, will quickly bring any rampant sweet tooth to heel, and from there, it can be retrained. Luckily, reducing sweet tastes is easier than it might sound as the taste receptors in our mouth and tongue adjust surprisingly quickly. You're talking weeks, not months, or years. All you have to do is try it.

7
Oily

Saturated fat was the nutritional folk devil of the second half of the 20th century. For 50 years, the dietetic establishment, first in the USA, then in the UK and worldwide, scapegoated it for obesity, heart disease, and stroke. Public health advice fuelled the panic, embedding saturated fat avoidance in 'healthy eating' guidelines. Because this dietary dogma was advanced with all the characteristic self-confidence of 'evidence-based' science, it became an unquestionable, unimpeachable orthodoxy, one that was recycled and diffused not only through all relevant government departments and health services, but also by the processed food industry, which enthusiastically adopted its new role as purveyor of supposedly healthier alternatives.

This casting of saturated fat as the dietary devil incarnate seemed counterintuitive to many. How could natural fats that had sustained populations for centuries – butter, ghee, suet, dripping, lard, chicken, duck, goose, palm and coconut fat – suddenly be so bad for us? Why would Mother Nature create such deviant fats to shorten the life expectancy of the human race?

There were mutinous mumblings in some quarters. Bored with recycling the same old scary story about how 'sat fat' (now abbreviated for speed of demonization) was killing us in droves, magazines eventually turned to quirky exceptions, notably the 'French paradox'. This term, coined by Dr Serge Renaud, director of public medical research at the French National Institute of Health and Medical Research in Lyon, captured the apparent contradiction that the French had a relatively low incidence of cardiovascular disease despite eating a diet rich in saturated fat. His observation was warmly received in food-loving, food-literate France; some years later he was awarded the Légion d'honneur. But in common with all those who dared to question the anti-sat fat dogma, Renaud's research was dismissed as dangerous heresy in other countries, especially those of a Presbyterian inclination, and the evilness of saturated fat was zealously propagated. This entrenched dogma was repeated so assiduously that it became the key fact that even the least nutritionally educated members of society had absorbed. Hard fats = bad fats. Liquid oils = good fats. That was all you needed to know.

Seeing how the nutritional script was unfolding, food manufacturers dropped solid saturated fats faster than a flaming chip pan, and switched production to oils rich in polyunsaturates, such as corn, soy, safflower, sunflower and oilseed rape. The dietetic fatwa on saturated fat was good for their bottom line: polyunsaturated oils were, and still are, much cheaper to buy than saturated fats. But they did have a downside. Unlike saturated fats, which are stable at room temperature, keep reasonably well, and are fairly tolerant of being heated, polyunsaturated oils are highly susceptible to deterioration. Light and heat have a devastating impact on their more sensitive chemical structure.

So although using vegetable oil high in polyunsaturates has been widely seen as a healthy choice, this is only half the story, as one oil company executive explains: 'If you heat it up, then you degrade it and create much more reactive substances than monounsaturated [the predominant fat in olive oil and many meats] or saturated fat.'

In an attempt to make polyunsaturate-rich oils more stable, oil suppliers adopted a technique known as hydrogenation, which had been developed for hardening soaps. Liquid oils were heated and combined with hydrogen atoms using a nickel catalyst. These oils, referred to as partially hydrogenated, did the job that manufacturers needed done. Hydrogenation acts as a preservative. The hardened oils stay fresher longer, giving products an accommodatingly long shelf life. Partially hydrogenated vegetable oils and fats became the mainstay of the processed food industry, for everything from margarine, salad dressings and sauces to pre-cooked chips, chicken nuggets, crisps and fish fingers.

Under pressure from the anti-sat fat lobby, fast food companies followed suit, bragging about their change to heart-healthy oils. The oily slide to jettison saturated fats even trickled down to chip shops. Where previously beef dripping had been the fat of choice, 'we fry in vegetable oil' banners appeared in windows. It seemed like a forward-thinking change to make, as one Scottish fish and chip shop owner recalls:

> I was aware of the reputation of fish and chips as an unhealthy food, so I thought, 'Let's try something different'. I decided to promote the change as a benefit, so I advertised in the local press that I was using an

> all-vegetable product, which was healthier. I did lose two customers who were diehard dripping users, but I gained so many people who wanted to try a vegetable product that my business has grown by 25%.

By the 1990s, however, the bad news about partially hydrogenated oils was seeping out, rather like a greasy stain that calls for a fresh change of clothes. It emerged that hydrogenation created 'trans fats', and these man-made fats were pretty deadly. Following the release of several scientific studies showing that eating trans fats increased the risk of developing heart disease, stroke and type 2 diabetes, health advocacy groups in the USA started campaigning for the food industry to remove them from their products.

At first, industrial food companies were in denial, hoping that these unsavoury revelations would melt away. They didn't. By 2002, the US government acknowledged for the first time that there was no safe level of trans fat, and that people should eat as little of it as possible. By 2006, it was mandatory to list trans fat on US food labels. Come 2010, reducing intake of trans fats was a key recommendation of the Dietary Guidelines for Americans. In the UK, the FSA took no such action, justifying its inaction on the basis that manufacturers were voluntarily removing trans fats from their products. In commercial terms, although they still linger on in products such as crackers, biscuits, cakes, frozen pies and frozen pizza, microwave popcorn, coffee creamers, and ready-to-use frostings, the writing is on the wall for trans fats on both sides of the Atlantic.

So in an echo of the flight from saturated fats, manufacturers who value their reputation have dumped, or are in the process of dumping, trans fats. Faithful to the anti-sat fat dogma, they continue to use polyunsaturate-rich oils, but now choose only the unhardened, non-hydrogenated sort – but this presents them with a number of technical challenges. Essentially, the less saturated fat is, the less stable it is, so non-hydrogenated oils are something of a nightmare to work with. 'For me, the biggest issue in frying today is the incorrect use of polyunsaturated oil for deep fat frying', says one oil company executive. 'It's pretty cheap. The downside is – and people don't realise it – it goes off faster [than saturated fat].'

So how does it 'go off' exactly? The first obvious consequence is flavour. When polyunsaturated oil degrades it quite quickly develops a distinctive taste and aroma that oil experts refer to as 'fishy'. If you have ever reheated deep-fried factory foods, such as hash browns or onion bhajis, that description might evoke some memories.

The next problem is that polyunsaturated oil builds up gunk, as this chemical company advice service explains:

> Over the past decade, as foodservice operators and food manufacturers have eliminated trans fats from their menus and food products, they have experienced some unexpected consequences from their use of zero trans fat oils. One such consequence is polymerisation, which causes gunk to form a coating on frying and manufacturing equipment. Polymerisation also can leave a film on kitchen and front-of-the-house surfaces that is both difficult and costly to remove.

Polymers are in the mist of oxidised fat that comes out of the deep-fat fryer, forming a sticky, varnish-like deposit on everything around – walls, work surfaces, utensils, workers' hair and clothing. Most of us will have inhaled polymers in takeaway and fast food restaurants, or from the heavy, smelly air that hangs around outside them.

A further problem is that aldehydes, the breakdown products from polyunsaturated fats, are much more reactive – so in effect, trouble-causing – than those of either saturated or monounsaturated fat. In fact, the toxicity of these aldehydes is well established in scientific literature: 'The geno- and cytotoxicity of these latter compounds [aldehydes] is well known and they have recently been thought to be responsible for several diseases, such as cancer, Alzheimer's and Parkinson's', one recent study concluded. We can ingest aldehydes either directly from the degraded oils by inhalation – a particular occupational hazard for factory workers – or by eating foods fried at high temperatures.

In a nutshell, although food manufacturers are gradually eliminating killer trans fats from their products, the polyunsaturate-rich vegetable oils they rely on still represent a Pandora's box of problems. Seeing trouble looming, suppliers of oils are now marketing a new wave of polyunsaturate-based vegetable oils that, wait for it, are said to have a healthier profile than their predecessors. Is this beginning to sound familiar?

The sales pitch this time round is that these latest oils are high in oleic fatty acids, also known as Omega-9s, (the dominant fat in olive oil), and lower in linolenic acid. The latter has the bad habit of decomposing during deep frying into acrolein, a pungent, possibly carcinogenic aldehyde compound that irritates the eyes and respiratory tract. 'Omega-9 oils are the next generation in healthier oils because of their unique health profile', Dow AgroSciences assures us. 'Our oils allow the foodservice and food processing industries to reduce 'bad' (trans and saturated) fats and increase good' (monounsaturated and polyunsaturated) fats in food products, making healthier options more readily available.' Déjà vu. Back to the script we have learnt by rote, that now familiar binary opposition between killer and saviour fats, and yet again, the actors playing the roles have been changed.

Still, surely anything that makes cooking oil more like olive oil has to represent progress? Sadly not. While the oleic acid in olive oil may be perfectly life-enhancing when it is anointing your mozzarella, tomato and basil salad, it behaves quite differently when heated up for deep frying. To be more specific, it produces breakdown products – oxidised monomeric triglycerides – that are absorbed in the human stomach and intestinal tract. These have been linked to cardiovascular disease and type 2 diabetes.

Of course any oil, however virgin and healthful at the outset, will come a cropper with overheating, and this is true whether you are frying in a domestic kitchen, a takeaway, or in a factory. The longer the oil is in use, the greater the presence of undesirable breakdown products. But in home cooking, oil is generally used once or twice, then discarded. On a factory scale, oils are used intensively over and over again, typically for anything from 7 up to 12 days; and remember that many food processing factories work round the clock. As one industry observer notes:

> In a commercial [factory] setting, it's a wonder that oils survive at all considering the ways in which they are abused. Large surface areas of industrial fryers expose the oil to air

> and oxidative stress. Accumulation of crumbs from cooked food further abuses the oil. High temperatures used in frying break down oil faster.

Food manufacturers often rely on methods as crude as colour change, or a weekly schedule, to determine when to change frying oil. Up-and-coming high oleic acid oils give them a lot more leeway because they hold up longer at higher temperatures, as one advocate for their deep-frying potential points out:

> These higher smoke-point [high oleic acid] oils extend use of frying oil without sacrificing taste or performance. Not only does this help maintain a consistent product, but fewer oil changes mean savings on labor and on the oil itself. Some high-oleic soybean oils can extend fry life two to three times longer than conventional versions.

Clearly, oils have to be tough as nails to withstand the rigours of commercial-scale deep frying. And in this respect, you can forget those produced by quaint traditional extraction methods, such as cold pressing; that's sissy stuff. Food manufacturers need battle-hardened marines that have survived an assault course even before they get to the factory.

This is why the oils that are destined for factory frying and fast food use are known as RBD, short for refined, bleached and deodorised. They owe their neutral flavour and prodigious keeping quality to a thoroughly industrial refining process. The oil seeds are crushed, and the oil is extracted using solvents, usually hexane. More chemicals are used to remove most (although not all) of the solvents; residues do remain. By this point in the refining process, some gummy stuff will have appeared in the oil, so it needs to be degummed, with the aid of either acids or enzymes. Hot by this point, the oil doesn't smell so good and will have darkened in colour, so it then has to be bleached using clay. Next up, it must be deodorised, which means heating it to a very high temperature at least twice. Put it this way, the RBD process produces oils that are hot and bothered, the very opposite of cold, unruffled and artisan.

Of course, when we buy cheap refined vegetable oil for home frying purposes, these are also RBD oils, but at least home cooks don't add anything further to them, unlike food manufacturers. To get the maximum longevity from their oils in the deep-fat fryer, food manufacturers and fast food outlets can add a number of 'improving agents' that extend the 'fry life', that is, delay the chemical degradation of the oil. First on the list of possibilities are antioxidants, basically preservatives by another name, such as citric acid, gallates, TBHQ (tert-butylhydroquinone), which is also used in varnishes and resins, and BHA (butylated hydroxyanisole). This last item 'is reasonably anticipated to be a human carcinogen'. It usually comes in a solution of propylene glycol (antifreeze) and is wonderfully user-friendly because it 'remains colourless even when heated at 194°C for one hour'. Next, an antifoaming agent might be added, such as polydimethylsiloxane (a type of silicon), along with an anti-spattering agent, such as lecithin. An emulsifier, such as mono- and diglycerides of fatty acids, can also go into the blend. Most commercial-scale fryers will also use mineral filters, such as silica, bentonite and perlite, to slow down the build-up of tacky, sticky deposits. As you will appreciate, there's more in industrial cooking oil than just straight oil, yet none of it appears on the label of the finished fried product – your packet of tortilla chips, your doughnut, your chicken Kiev – because they count as processing aids, not additives.

Another long-life frying medium coming into the frame for food manufacturers is EE – extruded expelled oil, usually from soya. More expensive, and still a minority choice, at first view it looks like a less chemical alternative to RBD oil. The oil seeds are squeezed through small metal holes, under high pressure and high temperature. But its main appeal to food manufacturers and fast food restaurants appears to be that it offers an exceptionally long fry life. As one US chef noted: 'We had been changing our frying oil every five to seven days. Suddenly we were able to go 12–14 days using the new [EE] oil.'

You can certainly see why food manufacturers might want to get away from industrially refined oils. The process creates a contaminant, 3-MCPD, linked with infertility in rats, suppression of immune function and possible carcinogenicity. The International Agency for Research on Cancer classifies it as a 'possible human carcinogen'. Nevertheless, the EU's Scientific Committee on Food has established a 'tolerable daily intake' for 3-MCPD. So what if there's another little dose of carcinogen in our food? The powers that be don't seem to be bothered. And if you happen to be a higher than average consumer of deep-fried foods, that's just your tough luck.

Whatever the oil of choice, the extreme heat and length of time required to fry certain popular foods creates another well-documented health hazard: acrylamide. This nerve poison causes cancer in animals and is classed by the US

Environmental Protection Agency as a 'probable carcinogen' in humans. In 2014, the European Food Safety Authority eventually concluded that acrylamide poses a bigger cancer risk to humans – particularly children – than it had previously thought. Up until then, it had taken the line that there was insufficient evidence available to determine the actual risk.

Crisps and chips have been identified as the biggest source of acrylamide in the British diet. In 2013, Bradford-based researchers – part of an international team studying the diet of pregnant women and newborns – concluded that women who eat foods high in acrylamide during pregnancy are more likely to produce babies with lower birth weights and smaller head circumferences. These birth outcomes have been linked to subsequent health problems, such as delayed development of the brain and nervous system. British babies had the highest levels of acrylamide of all the five European centres studied, almost twice the level of Danish babies, largely because their mothers share the national fondness for deep-fried chips and crisps.

Obviously, food manufacturers and fast food chains can't take all the blame for the UK's high acrylamide intake. Many home cooks use their own deep-fat fryer, although the widespread availability of pre-fried oven chips makes that piece of equipment increasingly redundant. But although acrylamide is found in homemade foods, international scientists studying the toxin for the EU's Heatox (Heat-Generated Food Toxicants) project, concluded that 'a large proportion of acrylamide intake comes from industrially-prepared food'. They pointed out that the amount of acrylamide we eat in home-cooked food is 'relatively small, when compared with industrially or restaurant-prepared foods'.

The sheer retail abundance of factory-fried products that few home cooks would ever attempt to make at home certainly spurs us on to eat more fried foods than we otherwise might, simply because they are so hassle-free. Frying crisps is not a core competence of the home cook, and why would you bother anyway, when crisps are probably the easiest food to buy in Britain? Where doesn't sell crisps? It is food manufacturing that makes high intakes of deep-fried products, such as crisps, possible.

Only the most devoted home cooks will go to the effort of breading a chicken breast or a piece of fish, first coating it with flour, then dipping it in eggs and breadcrumbs, then frying it. Very few domestic cooks will go to the bother of making a batter from scratch. But it is seductively easy these days just to pop a pre-battered or breadcrumbed meal in the microwave.

In fact, breadcrumbs and batters are a big feature of many processed foods. No wonder. They bulk out the more expensive ingredients. You can call something a chicken nugget even if its greasy, starchy jacket vastly outweighs the meagre quantity of mulched chicken meat within. As for breaded or battered scampi, that was always a licence to print money, a strategy for selling derisory amounts of blitzed-up prawn padded out by oily cladding.

Food manufacturers also find batters and crumb coatings useful because they reduce one of their perennial technical issues: excessive oil 'pick-up'. Here is the problem; when food is cooked in really fresh hot oil, the oil acts as a heat transfer agent, and there is no excessive absorption of oil into the food (pick-up). But as industrial food manufacturers use oils over and over again, the chemical and physical properties of the oil change, causing more oil to be absorbed. Never fazed, food manufacturers get round this challenge by creating an edible film around the food (turkey drummer, fish fillet, veggie burger, whatever) to bind in moisture. To do this job, they can turn to specially developed fish, meat and dairy proteins, sugar-based 'gelators', or hydrocolloids such as xanthan gum, konjac or HPMC ((hydroxypropyl)methyl cellulose). These gummy aids form a sticky barrier gel around the food and contribute greatly to its 'freeze-thaw' stability. In other words, the batter or crumb won't appear soggy and start coming away from the food when it is defrosted. A 'pre-dusting' in a chemically modified starch will also act, in food manufacturing language, as a 'texturiser', sealing in moisture and reducing 'blow-out' (when the food bursts out of its coating).

Somehow, the more you learn about commercial-scale deep frying, the less you feel like eating the resulting products, and to give full credit to the public health establishment in this regard, you have been warned. Most of us have heard the message that too many deep-fried foods are bad for our health, even if we tend to believe that saturated fat is the reason for the objection. But when polyunsaturate-rich oils are used to make non-fried products, in industrial baking for example, they are presented as nutritional saviours. The smoothest and most oleaginous of ambassadors for this proposition is margarine, or to give it its more bewitching modern title, low-fat spread. Low-fat spread is the family pet of the UK nutrition establishment, head prefect and hero product, an Achilles in the vanguard of the healthy eating charge. Its healthfulness is enshrined in government eating advice. The NHS even helps to sell the stuff: 'Butter is high in fat, so try to use it sparingly. Low-fat spreads can be used instead of butter', it tells us with great authority.

Actually, you'd think that the dietetic establishment might by now have become more circumspect in the advice it dispenses, given that for half a century, it promoted margarine spreads stiff with trans fats, which we now know to be decisive life-shorteners. In 1993, for instance, the leading 'heart-healthy' margarine contained 21% trans fats and 'normal' margarines were one-third trans fats. It is only in the last decade that manufacturers have begun reformulating their spreads with allegedly less damaging alternatives. But don't expect any mea culpa, no 'sorry, we got it wrong' statement from government nutrition gurus, or for that matter from the charities that become plump and lazy, recycling and disseminating tablets of nutritional wisdom dispensed from above. Instead, they have tried to bury that particular embarrassment.

While NHS guidelines now grudgingly acknowledge that 'consuming a diet high in trans fats can lead to high cholesterol levels in the blood, which can lead to health conditions, such as heart attacks, strokes and heart disease', a statement to minimise any alarm caused follows closely. 'However, most people in the UK don't eat a lot of trans fats. We eat about half the recommended maximum of trans fats on average, which is why the more commonly eaten saturated fat is considered a bigger health risk'. In other words, trans fats weren't and aren't a problem, but those deviant saturated fats devised by psychopathic Mother Nature are still the root of all evil. This continues to be the entrenched official nutrition gospel, even though in 2010, a major review of 21 scientific studies on fat stated that 'there is no significant evidence for concluding that saturated fat causes heart disease'. By 2014, the British Heart Foundation was still adhering to its anti-saturated fat doctrine after a systematic, wide-ranging study, funded by the foundation itself, examined 72 academic studies involving more than 600,000 participants, and found that saturated fat consumption was not associated with coronary disease risk.

For their part, manufacturers of spreads are keen to tell us, once again, that they are now using much healthier trans fat-free oils. Groundhog day. This time interesterified fats are presented as the heroes of the hour. But are they?

To make these interesterified fats, oil refiners rearrange the fatty acids in liquid oil at a high temperature, and under pressure, using enzymes or chemical catalysts. This changes the melting points and makes the resulting oils harder and more 'plastic' or malleable. Whether interesterified oils are any less lethal in health terms than the hydrogenated ones they are replacing remains to be seen, but already research studies are flagging up negative effects on blood glucose, insulin, immune function and liver enzymes in humans. As one group of researchers warns: 'More research is warranted to determine the appropriateness of interesterified fat consumption, particularly before it becomes insidiously embedded in the food supply similar to TFA [Trans Fatty Acids] and intake levels are achieved that compromise long-term health.' That sounds awfully like scientists saying: 'We made a big mistake with trans fats. Let's not make another one.'

Nevertheless, the dietetic establishment's evangelical enthusiasm for spreads, now made with RBD oils that have been interesterified, goes on unchecked. For instance, in 2014 the UK government Change4Life campaign, which is meant to be about urging citizens to make healthier food choices, asked: 'Why not swap butter in your mash for lower fat butters and spreads?' Anticipating groans and 'Do I have to?' reactions, it added chirpily: 'It will still be creamy and just as tasty.'

Really? Even margarine manufacturers never try to assert that spreads taste as good as butter. Wisely so: to do so is preposterous. Butter has an inimitable flavour, and is clean on the palate. Margarine spreads, on the other hand, leave a greasy coating on the roof of the mouth and taste of nothing pleasant. Yet switching from butter to margarine is a UK government-endorsed 'Smart Swap'. That our public health advisers never miss an opportunity to champion such a thoroughly artificial and fake food concoction speaks volumes about their failure to grasp the essentials of good food. But it does highlight their queasily close embrace of industrial food manufacturing, and all its dubious products.

If you think about it, margarine is an edible construction that owes its very existence to technology. It is a forced marriage of two cheap substances that won't naturally come together: oil – refined and processed out of all recognition – and water. This unwilling twosome is coerced into an alliance brokered by emulsifying additives. The resulting slippery sludge then needs to be coloured to be lifted out of murky greyness, flavoured to help us get it down our gullets, fortified with vitamins it lacks, and spiked with substances to stop it turning rancid. Is this *really* what we ought to be eating?

8

Flavoured

So accustomed are we to seeing that familiar word 'flavouring' on the ingredients lists of manufactured food, we have almost stopped noticing it. At one level, it is easily comprehensible: a substance that imparts flavour. At another level, the term is utterly opaque. What is flavouring actually? Is it animal, vegetable, mineral? How is it made? What is its composition? What does it look like? We swallow these mystery additives regularly in everything from crisps and drinks to ready meals and yogurts, yet most of us haven't a clue about them.

Because flavourings always sit so far down on the ingredients listing, we can be forgiven for assuming that they are just trivial little extras. Like a few last-minute drops of truffle oil on a painstaking risotto, we want to think that they are merely rounding off well-made food. But that perception couldn't be further from the truth. Although food manufacturers add flavourings to processed food in tiny quantities, they have a disproportionately transformative effect on them. In fact, they are the miraculous 'X factor' that makes countless manufactured foods possible. In the words of the flavouring company, Carotex: 'It is difficult to imagine how certain products would taste without flavours added in their production.' And why might that be? 'The technological processes of mass food production often result in loss of flavour and mouthfeel. To compensate for this, products are enriched with supplementary flavours.'

This circumspect language does not convey the full extent of food manufacturers' dependency on flavourings. Forget enrichment; that term implies that you are taking something that is well endowed with flavour in its own right, then improving it by adding something that further embellishes it. In the context of processed food, quite the opposite is the case. The hard fact of the matter is that the extreme temperatures and stress involved in industrial food manufacture do grievous bodily harm to natural ingredients, irrevocably damaging their intrinsic textures, flavours and aromas. Any casualties that aren't dead on the pavement after the brutal assault are left clinging on to life in a shaky, weakened, scarred, never-the-same-again state. They need help, and so added flavourings step in to boost them, additives that make it possible to sell the otherwise unsellable by conning us into thinking that food and drink tastes of something that it does not.

Although hoodwinking our taste buds is the prime driver for adding flavourings, their pivotal importance in food processing doesn't end there. Not only do they cover for a dearth of true taste, they also do the vital job of actively suppressing undesirable flavours and smells created by the manufacturing process. Carotex informs its manufacturer clients that its flavourings can be used 'as masking agents to cover any unwanted odours'. Flaverco, a company selling dairy flavourings 'with flavour strength up to 70 times that of cream and milk', explains to prospective customers that they are 'excellent at masking off flavours'. These 'off' tastes and smells are part and parcel of industrial food processing, a consequence of severe treatments that denature them – ultra-heat treatment, centrifugation, evaporation, deodorising, spray drying, sterilisation, pasteurisation, extrusion, for instance – or traces of chemical solvents and residual contaminants, such as heavy metals.

Flavourings also hide the jarring tastes of common processed food ingredients. For instance, the trendy sweetener stevia, artificial sweeteners, whey protein, and the salt substitute potassium chloride, all leave lingering bitter, metallic tastes. Soya protein and added vitamins trail astringency in their wake. The Butter Buds® company, whose quaintly folksy motto is 'Making the most of Mother Nature', sells its dairy flavourings to 'round out harsh notes', for which read residual taints lingering on from the production process that would offend the olfactory system. Symrise is another company active in the flavour-masking field that offers manufacturers 'customised masking solutions for tastes you want to hide'. It says that its 'flavor development expertise, creative problem-solving skills and technological toolbox of masking agents' can help manufacturers overcome 'undesirable sensory perceptions, avoid troublesome off-flavors', and 'suppress off-notes while simultaneously increasing flavor impact'. As you can see, in food manufacturing, getting rid of unpalatable tastes and reeks is almost as much of a preoccupation as adding in desirable ones.

Flavourings deceive our taste buds and disguise the stink of industrial food manufacture, but they also perform a purely financial function: they are cheap, and so make it possible for manufacturers to use less of something more expensive. As the cost of real food ingredients steadily mounts, manufacturers have a strong financial incentive to bump up their use of flavourings. Less cheese, more cheese flavouring, less lemon juice, more lemon flavouring, less beef, more beef flavouring, and so on. It's only business sense.

Kalsec®, a company very active in flavouring supply, offers this example of just how profitable dialogue between food industry chemists ('flavourists' as they prefer to be known) and manufacturers can be:

> A leading manufacturer of private label [branded] foods met our team at an industry trade show. They inquired about cost savings for one of their condiment products. Following up with this customer immediately after the show, Kalsec®'s team went to work. While cost savings was the goal, it was equally important to match the existing flavor profile of this product. The Kalsec® Application Team analysed the product and returned within two weeks with a matching profile for bench scale testing. In collaboration with the Kalsec® team, the private label company made minor tweaks in the formulation and a successful liquid alternative was developed. This condiment was now ready for store shelves at a considerable savings and with a timely turnaround.

'Considerable saving' is a term guaranteed to prick up the ears of food manufacturers, and flavourings make it possible to put an appealing ingredient on a product label, but use very little of it. An industry flavour chemist offers the example of the recently fashionable, and very expensive, açai berry:

> Instead of adding açai juice to a dairy beverage, a natural açai [flavouring] could be added, which consists of açai extracts and natural aroma materials to mimic açai taste. A flavor is preferred, because the overall taste nuance can be adjusted – fresh versus fruity, versus jammy or cooked. The flavor also allows for an increased shelf life, provides ease of use and decreases cost.

Put it this way, flavourings may be small in bulk, but they are mighty and multi-tasking in effect. Simulation, modification, masking, that's the very essence of flavouring, as one flavour chemist summarises:

> Flavors are used to impart or simulate a taste characteristic of choice, to modify a flavor that is already present, to maintain the flavor character after processing or to mask some undesirable flavor to increase consumer acceptance.

So much research and development goes into formulating flavourings that it's hard for food manufacturers to keep up to speed with the technology. The lists, portfolios, catalogues and 'flavour libraries' of flavouring companies are lengthy, and couched in terminology that is as slippery as an eel. They include flavour components, flavour emulsions, flavour boosters, recovery flavourings, concentrated and non-concentrated flavourings, replacer flavourings, heat management flavourings, bitterness blockers, fantasy flavourings, flavour precursors, soy suppressors, top-notes, long flavourings, reaction flavourings and sensation flavourings. The latter are evidently designed to thrill the palate. Some companies try helpfully to explain to their customers the function of the various options. The 'flavour solution' categories used by Comax, for instance, include 'acid masking flavours, mouth-feel [mouth filling] flavours, debitterising flavours, sweetness enhancing flavours, fat replacing flavours, fried note flavours, cooling flavours, salt enhancing flavours', and last but not least, 'salivation enhancers'. Just reading this classification makes you want to lick your lips.

If food manufacturers need help to keep abreast of the latest innovations in the flavouring field, and make their selection from literally thousands of flavouring products that enable a dizzying number of flavour permutations, what should an industry outsider make of them all?

When you open the door onto food industry flavourings, you walk into a most original and downright ingenious grand bazaar of man-made smells and tastes. To get our bearings, most of us will seek out those we know, old stalwarts like peppermint. But then the eclectic selection spins off like a Catherine wheel in all directions, and the further into this odiferous marketplace we go, the more fantastical, hallucinogenic and positively surreal those flavourings become.

The selection begins with a comprehensive list of fruit flavourings, everything from passion fruit and pitahaya, through to peach and pomegranate, with multiple cultivars represented, so you don't just get raspberry flavouring, you also get black raspberry flavouring. There is an entire family of grape flavourings alone – Arkadia, Concorde, Isabella, Muscat and more. The foraging section includes sea buck-thorn, truffle and rosehip flavourings. In the carvery, there are 'hamburger spice', fried chicken, smoked salmon, Serrano ham, Polish ham, bacon, roasted pork, boiled pork, beef, barbecue, chicken bouillon and 'herb-crusted ham' flavourings. Various smoke flavourings (mesquite, hickory, beech, oak, applewood) jostle for attention next to roast chicken, pit-roasted pork, Arabian burger flavourings and a 'deliciously slow roasted prime rib of beef' variant developed to 'give your products that special authenticity note'. Not just any old flavouring then, but a special, slow-roasted flavouring from a named butcher's cut. Bear in mind that many flavourings, such as Parma ham, sourdough bread and quince, are clearly designed for use in up-market products, items for which you'll pay a premium at the delicatessen.

Fishy flavourings are represented en masse: anchovy, concentrated clam, crab, generic 'seafood', scallop and a whole shoal more. The vegetables and herbs section in the flavourings emporium is stacked to the roof with garlic, asparagus, potato, spring onion, marjoram, tomato, celery, onion, shallot, cucumber, and every other vegetable you can think of, in various cooked (char-grilled, roasted, sun-dried) and raw states.

By way of spices and condiments, ketchup, Cajun, pimento, allspice, anise, black pepper, Jamaican jerk, Dijon mustard, Worcestershire sauce, Kimchi and gingerbread flavourings are just a drop in an ocean of possibility. There are pistachio, walnut, chestnut, peanut, macadamia, sesame, coconut and coconut water flavourings, pesto and pizza flavourings a go-go. Vanilla offers a whole tribe: Tahitian, Mexican, vanilla 'cream'. Honey represents another family tree with several branches: clover, acacia, lavender, pine, chestnut, thyme. The dairy department groans with cheesecake, cream, mascarpone, tiramisu, Gorgonzola, feta, ricotta,

Emmental, mozzarella, goat's cheese, buttermilk and yogurt flavourings.

Flavourings also come as custom-made blends tailored to one product. A biscuit manufacturer can source, for instance, a 'custard cream' flavouring, an 'oatmeal cookie enhancer', or a 'bun spice' flavouring. A caterer or ready meals company can turn some pre-sliced frozen potatoes into a plausibly authentic and aspirational tartiflette – the classic Savoyarde dish – by merely adding some powdered tartiflette flavouring 'prepared from bacon notes, Reblochon and cooked onions with crème fraiche'. A lazy chef can use a carbonara flavouring powder: 'This 100% natural flavour will give a desired taste of Parmesan, bacon and crème fraiche to food creations'. For the romantic and naive, there are long, lyrical, composite flavourings, such as coconut chocolate almond vanilla, and white chocolate macadamia nut, or Crazy Caprese Mediterranean blend.

From Polynesian plum, pina colada, prickly pear and pumpkin pie to banana, beer, butterscotch and broccoli, no flavour, however notional, appears to be beyond the endeavour of flavour engineers. The sheer scale and ambition of their mission is so uncoupled from the realm of fact that it takes the breath away. Flavour chemists clearly believe that there is no flavour in nature that they cannot capture. Their confidence in their trade is absolute. According to FlavorFacts, an industry body:

> Flavorists work in a combined field of art and science, using a 'flavor palette' the same way a painter uses color or a sculptor uses texture. There are a range of flavor ingredients that impart tastes (sweet, sour, salty, bitter, and

> savory), smells, and physical traits ('heat' and 'cold'), and we experience these flavors and traits at different points while we eat. Flavorists refer to these as 'notes,' with the 'top note' being the first thing you taste, and the 'bottom note,' the last. Flavorists can mix and match from their palette to make a seemingly unlimited number of flavor combinations.

But these chemists who are playing around with our taste buds need a reality check. Whether 'natural' or artificial, flavourings never manage to replicate the real thing. A croissant made with butter flavouring and margarine doesn't taste the same as one made with real butter. Pistachio ice cream made with pistachio flavouring can never be confused with one made with a generous quantity of crushed fresh nuts. A drink concocted with lime flavouring is not at all like one made with zingy fresh lime juice. This much is apparent to anyone who eats real food and therefore has benchmark natural flavours against which to judge the man-made pretenders.

Of course, flavour chemists don't see taste that way. For them, any natural flavour is nothing more or less than an assembly of volatile chemicals, such as phenols, terpenes and esters, which excite the nose and activate the taste buds. Once the most dominant of these heady compounds has been isolated, and their chemical structure fathomed, they can then be synthesised to produce flavourings that capture their essence. Find them, name them, copy them – what could be simpler?

Currently, there is a grand total of 2,500 'approved flavouring substances' or aromatic chemicals that can be legally used to flavour food in Europe. Four hundred of these are under evaluation for safety, and so could eventually be removed. This process takes years, if not decades. The list features substances such as 1-isopropyl-4-methylbenzene, 2,6-dimethylocta-2,4,6-triene, 2-methyl-1-phenylpropan-2-ol, cyclohexanol, 3-(1-menthoxy)propane-1,2-diol, 9-octadecenal, 1-isopentyloxy-1-propoxyethane, 3,4-dihydroxybenzoic acid, cinnamyl butyrate, 3-[(4-amino-2,2-dioxido-1H-2,1,3-benzothiadiazin-5-yl)oxy]-2,2-dimethyl-N-propylpropanamide, lenthionine, and another 2,490 of that ilk.

The approved list might not whet the appetite, yet it catalogues some of the chemical components of many mouthwatering flavours. Allyl hexanoate, for instance, smells like pineapple, ethyl decadienoate like pears, while benzaldehyde and limonene conjure up bitter almond and orange, respectively. In the flavourist's jargon, they are 'tastants', chemicals that stimulate the sensory cells in our taste buds. Chemicals such as these are the building blocks from which food industry chemists construct the flavourings that end up in our food and drink. A typical strawberry flavouring for a milk shake, for example, is composed of around 50 such chemicals. 'We can get compounds like hydrogen sulfide and dimethyl sulfide that generate the sulfuric flavor of aged Cheddar, or a mixture of esters – ethyl benzoate, ethyl butyrate, etc. – that give off a fruity flavor like in Parmesan', one 'sensory coordinator' explains. Dimethyl sulfide, 2-acetyl-1-pyrroline and 2-acetyl-2-thiazoline, for example, evoke cooked flavours, whereas strong, nutty flavours might come from 2- and 3-methylbutanal. Amyl acetate flags up banana, benzaldehyde does the same for cherry.

If creating flavourings was only a matter of mix and match, or cut and paste, then flavourists would be redundant in their droves overnight, but aping the flavours of the natural world is hard. Nature's flavours are intricate, and composed of not one but many of these aromatic chemicals. In a high-grown coffee, for instance, there are hundreds of flavour notes, including berry, citrus and jasmine. In cocoa, more than 600 flavours have so far been identified. To date, some 10,000 flavours have been identified in nature, and it's a dead cert that there are many more just waiting to be discovered.

Any natural flavour is an elaborate thing, with legions of odoriferous chemicals acting in synergy to create that distinctive taste and fragrance fingerprint. It's one thing to be able to identify the major chemicals that underpin a certain flavour and aroma, quite another to formulate a flavouring that does justice to the sheer complexity and well-ordered intelligence of the real thing. Flavour engineers can tinker all they like with the proportions and combinations of chemicals to come up with more convincingly real flavours, but they can only get so close.

A further stumbling block in flavour construction, or 'taste modulation' as the trade likes to call it, is that the flavours in natural food come all wrapped up in natural macro- and micronutrients – proteins, fats, carbohydrates, vitamins, minerals – that taste good. Natural foods are holistically conceived packages, with every element supporting several more and contributing to the common good. But in industrial food manufacture, many of the bulk ingredients in the recipe are already so corrupted and traduced by excessive processing – industrially refined vegetable oil, lifeless, nutritionally denuded bulk starches and fillers, for instance – that they bring precious little to the table in taste terms, or worse, make everything taste bad.

Low-fat products represent a particularly tough challenge for flavour chemists. Many flavours are lipophilic, that is, they are most concentrated in fat. Fat is flavour's friend, so if manufacturers decrease the fat in foods, flavour release happens more quickly and dissipates faster in the mouth. Less fat also diminishes creaminess, smoothness and viscosity. This is why low-fat milk doesn't taste as good as full-fat. Manufacturers also like to earn brownie points by reducing levels of sugar and salt in their products, but this results in a taste gap that flavouring helps to hide. And while real flavours fade or intensify over time, man-made flavourings maintain the same profile right up until the 'use-by' or 'best before' date. In the words of one flavour chemist, a flavouring must 'withstand whatever process it faces and [can] deliver the character you want over the life of the product'.

The task of the flavour chemists then, is not so much to concoct a chemical blend that has the refinement of the real thing, but to come up with a larger-than-life flavouring, a ramped-up version of reality that's fit for the job of disguising the vapidity of other industrialised ingredients.

So although the chemical industry is keenly focused on capturing and reproducing natural flavours, it is embarked on an impossible mission. At best, its efforts are akin to an amateurish counterfeiter's maladroit copy of a work of art. Others are so patently fake they are laughable; about as authentic as a mouthful of scented candle or whiff of air freshener. Indeed, candles, air fresheners and processed food flavourings can have aromatic chemicals in common.

Those people most preoccupied with avoiding the products of the processed food industry may draw the conclusion that it is best to avoid anything with the word 'flavouring' on the label, even if that means only eating plain salted crisps, and avoiding any beverage that has the weasel word 'drink' (code for 'with flavouring') in its name, but many more of us seek refuge in the cosseting adjective 'natural'. Natural flavouring sounds like a reasonable compromise, implying some sort of qualitative difference. If only. Even FlavorFacts, a promotional body of the flavouring industry, squashes that illusion: 'There isn't much difference in the chemical compositions of natural and artificial flavorings', it says. How can this be?

Natural and artificial flavourings do have a different genesis. Natural flavourings must be made from flavours chemically extracted from natural sources – plants, minerals and animals – just as you might expect. Artificial flavourings, on the other hand, are born in the laboratory.

There are two sorts of artificial flavourings. 'Nature identical' flavourings have the same chemical formula as their natural model, but are synthesised from chemicals. For example, Citral, or to give it its chemical name, 3,7-dimethyl-2,6-octadienal, has a strong lemon zest aroma, and whether it is distilled from lemon grass oil, or chemically synthesised in the lab, it has the same molecular structure. A wholly 'artificial' flavouring, on the other hand, does not come from natural aromatic materials, and its chemical structure is not found anywhere in nature.

A classic example here is the artificial vanilla flavouring, ethyl vanillin. Probably the most extensively used flavouring in food manufacture, its cloying, heavy-handed faux vanilla presence finds its way into cakes, biscuits, sweets and ice cream. This artificial vanillin is usually chemically synthesised from sawdust, petrochemicals or wood pulp, with not a vanilla pod in sight. But it gives manufacturers more bang for their bucks, being 'roughly three times more taste-intensive' and much less costly than real vanilla.

If the distinction between natural and artificial flavourings seem clear enough, if not crystal clear, be prepared to be confused, or even bemused, by this further distinction in the 'natural' flavouring category. Food manufacturers get to choose from three kinds of 'natural' flavouring: FTNSs, FTNFs and WONFs. They themselves bandy these acronyms around freely, but even in their unabbreviated form they don't ring a bell with the rest of us. And why should they? You won't see them on ingredients listings.

FTNS stands for 'From The Named Source', so a basil FTNS will have started out with real basil in some form – probably dehydrated and frozen – while an artificial basil flavouring will never have seen a leaf of the pungent herb. FTNF stands for 'From The Named Fruit'; such flavourings are particularly marketed as useful 'add-backs' for fruit juices to 'replace' the aromas of the fruit that have been destroyed in the production process.

WONF, which stands for 'With Other Natural Flavourings', is a trickier concept. Although these are sold by one name – blackcurrant, vanilla, hazelnut, cranberry, or whatever – such flavourings have been blended or 'enhanced', as the industry diplomatically puts it, with a mixture of other natural flavourings. To a member of the public looking at the ingredients list on a 'black cherry ice cream' for instance, the difference is far from obvious. Unless the label reads 'natural black cherry flavouring', there will certainly be other flavourings swirling around in the tub. Even when a flavouring is a FTNF, and described, for example, as 'natural black cherry flavouring', five per cent of it can come from chemicals not found in cherries to 'standardise' the taste.

At one trade show, I was given a sensory tutorial on natural honey flavourings at the stand of a company known for its cutting-edge products. Out from a locked drawer came diminutive phials of clear liquid. My tutor dipped those little flexible cardboard strips used at perfume counters into the liquid then wafted them under my nose. Had I been asked to identify them blind, I would probably have correctly plumped for honey, but I would have been unable to differentiate between the natural honey flavouring and the WONF version. But the weird and instructive thing about this experience was that although these heady clear substances made me recall honey, they were like no honey I have ever smelt or tasted. Rather, they reminded me of those scratch-and-sniff games where children are encouraged to identify an odour. They were bigged-up, exaggerated presences, and being around them was like being stuck in the front row of an opera where you can't help noticing the thickness of the singers' make-up.

The naturalness of 'natural' flavourings becomes even more debatable when you consider how they are made. When pressed to give examples of the methods used, flavour companies volunteer time-honoured methods, such as distillation and infusion, which evoke images redolent of Patrick Suskind's fragrant novel, *Perfume*. But the processes permitted for making natural flavourings are considerably broader, and more hi-tech, than such examples might lead you to believe.

In European law, a 'natural flavouring substance' can be obtained:

> by appropriate physical, enzymatic or microbiological processes from material of vegetable, animal or microbiological origin either in the raw state or after processing for human consumption by one or more of the traditional food preparation processes listed.

So making natural flavourings can include using microorganisms, such as bacteria, advanced fermentation techniques that involve genetic modification, and enzymes to speed up the chemical process. For instance, modern biotechnology can create a 'natural' mature cheese flavouring by blending young, immature cheese with enzymes (lipases or proteases) that intensify the cheese flavour until it reaches 'maturity' – within 24 to 72 hours. This mature cheese flavouring is then heat treated to halt enzymatic activity. Hey presto, mature-tasting cheese in days, not months. By comparison, traditional Cheddar is not considered truly mature until it has spent from nine to 24 months in the maturing room.

The production method for making natural flavourings can also entail extraction using solvents – propane, butane, methyl acetate, ethanol, acetone, nitrous oxide, hexane, ethyl methyl ketone, dichloromethane, propan-2-ol, diethyl ether, butan-1-ol, propan-1-ol and 1,1,1,2-tetrafluoroethane are all considered suitable for this purpose. Such solvents, we are assured, must be used 'in compliance with good manufacturing practice' and any residues or derivatives left in the flavouring must be 'technically unavoidable' and in quantities that present 'no danger to human health'. It's quite clear, however, that in some circumstances, flavouring chemicals can be a health hazard, as the US Government's Centers for Disease Control and Prevention (CDC) points out:

> Flavoring chemicals are very volatile, so they evaporate into the air from their liquid or solid form and can be easily inhaled. They can also be inhaled in the form of a powder if airborne dust is created in the production process. Many of these chemicals are highly irritating to the eyes, respiratory tract, and skin.

We're not just talking the odd sneeze here. As the CDC notes, exposure to flavourings is known to have caused severe lung disease in some workers routinely exposed to them. In fact, respiratory problems are a known occupational hazard for those whose job is on the flavouring line of crisp, popcorn and pretzel factories. And if exposure to flavourings can have such damaging effects on the people who work with them, what might it do in the long term to those who consume food and drink containing them? As always, the official line – that flavourings pose no risk to human health when ingested in small quantities – is scarcely reassuring. Safe limits for consumption of flavourings are based on statistical assumptions, often provided by companies who make food additives. And although they can refer to a long list of official risk assessments for individual additives, no independent regulatory body appears to be researching the potential cocktail effect of such additives on people who consume large quantities of processed food. Yet, as the CDC acknowledges, 'much remains unknown regarding the toxicity of flavoring-related chemicals'.

Consumers in Europe are gradually becoming as suspicious of the word 'flavouring' as they are of the word 'colouring'. In Germany in 2013, the highly respected consumer protection group, Stiftung Warentest (the German equivalent of Which?) was taken to court by the leading German chocolate brand, Ritter Sport, for suggesting that the vanilla flavouring in its hazelnut chocolate bars was not truly natural because it was made using chemicals. Ritter Sport won an injunction against Stiftung Warentest, but this high-profile dispute put the 'realness' of natural flavourings in the spotlight and left many German consumers wondering if, in practical terms, there is any significant difference between artificial and natural flavourings.

Anticipating a time when the term 'flavouring' might become irredeemably discredited – whether prefixed by natural or not – the food manufacturing industry is quite keen to elbow that troublesome word off its labels. So the push is on to replace flavourings with products that also enhance taste, but have less unsettling names. Two legal terms have now been established for these: 'flavouring preparations' and 'foods with flavouring properties'. These shiny new categories of up-and-coming flavour boosters include substances referred to on the ingredients list as 'natural extracts' and 'natural concentrates', which sound like something you'd eat on a yoga retreat. Where once your lunchtime couscous salad, prawn mayo sandwich and diet lemonade would have had 'flavouring' on the label, extracts and concentrates increasingly replace it. Move over lemon flavouring, and let's hear it for lemon juice extract or concentrate. But as the European Flavouring Association makes clear, these preparations can be produced using the same techniques as natural flavourings, 'from plant, animal or microbiological source materials by means of physical or biotechnological [GM] production processes'. So, this apparent move into naturalness isn't quite as decisive as we'd like to think.

To be fair, most of us would probably prefer, for instance, that an intensely savoury, meaty, added 'umami' taste came from yeast extract – a food with flavouring properties – rather than from MSG, the controversial artificial flavouring, linked with allergic reactions. But the rationale for adding flavours, whether that's in the form of natural or artificial flavourings, flavouring preparations, or foods with flavouring properties, is identical: they create a fake taste.

Ironically, European law is quite pernickety on fakery. It says:

> Flavourings should, in particular, not be used in a way as to mislead the consumer about issues related to, amongst other things, the nature, freshness, quality of ingredients used, the naturalness of a product or of the production process, or the nutritional quality of the product.

Excuse me, but isn't misleading the consumer precisely what added flavour is all about?

9
Coloured

Lack of colour is not a problem in natural food. Creamy white cauliflower, verdant peas, crimson raspberries, purple plums, shell-pink crab, garnet meat, eau de Nil fennel, ruby redcurrants, orange mussels, ecru oats, ochre turmeric, mossy-veined blue cheese, burgundy pomegranate, mercury-black rice, carnelian tuna, sunny lemon and many, many more – the palette of food colours used in nature is boundless, full of nuances, and profoundly beautiful.

These colours make natural food look appetising. This is why, whenever manufacturers want to sell us something, they make a point of putting an enticing picture of fresh food in its whole, unprocessed state on the label. It's the reason why soft drinks claiming to bear some relationship to oranges come plastered with images of the fresh fruit, even when they contain precious little of it.

Natural food has no less alluring colour when it's cooked. There's glamour in the brick-red oil bubbling up through the creamy, gratinated crust of a lasagne, lustre in blanched spring greens anointed in melted butter, pearliness in celeriac purée, amber sheen in caramelised apples on a tarte Tatin, a vivacity to hot blueberries staining a golden crumble. Nature's colour chart sells millions of recipe books illustrated with food photography because its bright visual diversity whets our appetites, without any retouching or colour enhancement.

But food manufacturers have a big issue with colour, a problem made explicit in the colouring guidelines issued to the food industry by the UK's FSA:

> Many raw foods such as fruit and vegetables have a bright attractive colour. However, the colour of some foods is reduced during food processing. Other foods such as confectionery items and flavoured soft drinks would be grey or colourless if colour was not added to them during the manufacturing process.

This cool executive summary is a strategic understatement. The industrial manufacturing process strips food of its pigments, spewing out lifeless, ashen, washed-out tones. If we saw it looking like this, we wouldn't want to eat it. Our brains wouldn't signal to us that we were seeing food. Perhaps we aren't.

Added colour is all-important in manufactured food, not only because it improves its dismal appearance, but also because it tricks us on flavour. The FSA explains how this sleight of hand works:

> The colour of food is important for consumers as it is the first characteristic to be noticed and one of the main ways of visually assessing a food before it is consumed. The perceived colour provides an indication of the expected taste of a food. If the flavour of a food product is inconsistent with the colour, the flavour can often be perceived

> incorrectly; for example an orange-flavoured drink coloured green could be perceived to taste of lime.

In other words, added colour cons us into thinking that processed food tastes of something that it doesn't, and primes us visually for the kind of flavour to expect, a party trick that helps cover up its yawning taste deficit. There is also a plausible theory that added colour provides a contextual cue to eat more. Brian Wansink, a professor of marketing and nutritional science, says: 'People eat with their eyes, and their eyes trick their stomachs. If we think there's more variety in a candy dish or on a buffet table, we will eat more. The more colors we see, the more we eat.'

While most of us can figure out that radiant sweets and lurid fizzy drinks must owe their gaudy hue to some sort of colorant, the general creep of added colour into thousands of everyday products largely passes us by. Yet imposter colours are in our sandwich fillers, soups, salads and sauces, in breads, biscuits and brioche, in fish, cheeses, meats and margarines. A dash of red makes pasta sauce look as if it contains more tomato than it really does. Just a hint of yellow mixed with orange makes anaemic waffles look deliciously bronzed. A smidgen of brown gives watery, starchy gravy in a ready-meal sausage hotpot a wholly misleading slow-cooked, concentrated appearance. The addition of green disguises the greyness of tinned peas.

It is no exaggeration to say that certain types of processed food would be unsellable without added colouring. A case in point is surimi, the heavily processed, minced fish protein that is used to imitate fresh prawns or crabmeat. This substance makes a frequent appearance in seafood hotpots served by Asian restaurants. It also turns up regularly buried in the centre of your sushi rolls, the sort you might pick up in supermarkets and takeaways, without closely examining the label. A range of red colourings give the grey fish protein mulch a pretty shrimp-pink hue. White colourings, such as calcium carbonate and titanium dioxide, endow it with the pearly whiteness of fresh crab claw meat.

From the late 1980s, concerns about colourings became the standard-bearer for a mounting critique of industrialised food. Following the publication in 1989 of Maurice Hanssen's influential book, *E for Additives*, public suspicion about food crystallised around them. Food campaigners picked up on research that suggested some of the most commonly used food colours could have adverse health effects, notably in children, the prime consumers of highly coloured products. Anecdotes circulated of toddlers who all but climbed the walls after sucking on orange lollies, or threw the most awful tantrums after eating strawberry jelly at a birthday party.

Food manufacturers hate their products being put in the spotlight; it's tricky when people start scrutinising ingredients and asking difficult questions. But rather than put a head above the parapet, they rely on our food regulators to fight their corner for them. By 2000, when the FSA was set up in response to calls for an independent food watchdog, it showed no particular appetite for tackling health issues around food colourings, but a turning point came in 2004 when a team of researchers from Southampton University concluded that six colours, used extensively in popular children's food, in combination with the preservative sodium benzoate, were causing hyperactivity and allergies in toddlers.

The colourings in question – sunset yellow (E110), quinoline yellow (E104), allura red (E129), carmoisine (E122), tartrazine (E102) and ponceau 4R (E124) – have subsequently gained notoriety as the 'Southampton Six'. These thoroughly artificial, chemically synthesised colours can contain toxins such as mercury and lead. Like many other food colourings, they also have many other industrial uses apart from food processing: textile colorants, paints, printing inks, varnishes, plastics, and crayons.

Presented with the Southampton findings, the FSA stepped in with reassuring words, as is its custom: 'All additives must pass strict safety checks before they can be used in foods and if any new evidence were to emerge from this or other work their safety would be reviewed.' However, the agency did fund the Southampton team to carry out further research. Three years later, the team came back with a second, more extensive study, published in *The Lancet*, one that is difficult to ignore. It studied 900 three- to nine-year-olds, and demonstrated a persuasive link between the consumption of these artificial colours and increased hyperactivity (attention deficit hyperactivity disorder).

Faced with a scientific study that it had to admit was of the highest quality, the FSA advised parents of children showing signs of hyperactivity to avoid giving them food and drink that contained the 'Southampton Six' colours, and encouraged food manufacturers to stop using the colours voluntarily. By 2010, under pressure from food campaigners, the UK had to go along with an EU-wide compulsory warning, instigated by the European Food Standards Agency, that any food and drink containing any of the six offenders must carry the health warning: 'May have an adverse effect on activity and attention in children.' A killer phrase, fit to stop even the most laid-back parents in their tracks. As one flavour company executive put it: 'Consumers are increasingly aware of the potential health risks associated with the consumption of artificial colours. These risks received substantiation with the decision by the European Food Standards Agency to force labelling on the "Southampton Six".'

In the UK, post the 'Southampton Six', food manufacturers began reformulating products, replacing artificial chemical colours with those that could legally be described comfortingly as 'natural'. Soft drinks were first in line. Asda, for instance, replaced the carmoisine in its cherryade, while Tizer removed ponceau 4R and sunset yellow, indicative of a widespread industry shift. Supermarkets demanded that their manufacturers remove any of the 'Southampton Six' colours from products such as ready-meal curries and curry sauces. Tandoori paste, for instance, owed its bright red colour to the inclusion of either allura red, carmoisine or ponceau 4R, sometimes combined with sunset yellow.

Food and drink manufacturers grumbled about the technical problems of swapping to 'natural' colourings. These are more inclined to bleed into one another, or look hazy. They aren't as intense as artificial ones, so manufacturers need to use more of them, and they are more prone to fading, so have a shorter shelf life. They are also more likely to form an oily ring in necks of bottles of coloured drinks. But it was an unstoppable tide; by 2011, global sales of 'natural' colourings outstripped those of artificial ones. Now, products containing the 'Southampton Six' have effectively been relegated to the food industry sin bin, and become an emblem for precisely the sort of product that anyone remotely informed will want to avoid: the worst sorts of fizzy drinks, the ghastliest gummy sweets. Under pressure from their customers, supermarkets can't get lines with artificial colourings off their shelves fast enough. M&S, for example, boasts that 99% of its food is free from artificial colours.

But all this activity leaves one very obvious question unanswered: if the 'Southampton Six' caused adverse reactions, what about all the other E number colours? Might they be as bad?

Now that's a very pertinent question, because these dyes aren't the only colours with persistent safety issues hanging over them. Artificial caramels, the sort used in cola, or to make muffins look more chocolatey, or to give meat an inviting roasted appearance, are a case in point. These are formulated by heating sugars, such as fructose, invert sugar or sucrose, and chemically modifying them, using acids, alkalis, or salts, so triggering a chemical reaction that produces the desired brown effect.

This class of brown colourings known as E150 in Europe, has been given 'generally regarded as safe' status by food regulators, provided we don't consume more than the specified 'acceptable daily intake', but this limit was calculated back in 1985, when we consumed much less food and drink containing caramel than we do now. Furthermore, it was based on safety-testing data presented by the caramel-colouring industry itself, in the shape of a body known as the European Technical Caramel Association (EUTECA), which describes its purpose as follows:

> EUTECA's mission is to improve general knowledge about caramel colour and its benefits, and to deliver factual information about caramel colour to European authorities, other bodies such as the Codex Alimentarius [an intergovernmental body that sets global food standards], and the general public, e.g. consumers or journalists.

Bluntly, EUTECA is a lobbyist for global food-additive companies with a vested interest in seeing their products commercialised, an organisation that knocks on the doors of regulators and arms them with a prêt-a-porter dossier to show that its members' products are safe. But prominent independent food groups don't accept that they are indeed safe, and are concerned that the ammonia sulfite process, used to make colouring for some colas, may form carcinogens. In the USA, cola brands have reformulated their drinks to remove the most controversial of these caramel colourings. In the UK, however, cola recipes remain unchanged as the European Food Safety Authority found that the original formulation does not pose a health risk to humans.

Like caramel, titanium dioxide E171 is another colouring in common use that is dogged by persistent health fears. Extracted from mineral ores, it makes hard shell chewing gums snowy white, and provides a base coat for coated sweets that allows the top colour to stand out. The base coat analogy is apt: titanium dioxide is also used to make paint. Described by one colour company representative as 'very cheap and very white', titanium dioxide is, according to the European Food Safety Authority, which is meant to be up-to-speed on these things, perfectly safe. It says: 'We are not aware of any scientific data supporting possible carcinogenic effects of oral exposure to titanium dioxide.' This colouring has, however, been classified by the International Agency for Research on Cancer as 'possibly carcinogenic to humans', and one study has suggested a link to Crohn's disease. In 2013 a spokesman for Beneo, a prominent food ingredients company, was heavily promoting its alternative to titanium dioxide in the trade press on the grounds that the latter had been 'flagged up as a possible cancer risk'.

One's instinct is to applaud the more forward-thinking food manufacturers who ditch colourings that have a question mark hanging over them long before any regulator gets around to making them do so, particularly if they then substitute them with something considered to be more natural. But that last word means different things to different people. Unfortunately for consumers who crave cut and dried information about food, but happily for food manufacturers who prefer a lot of wiggle room, there is no legal distinction in the EU between synthetic colours and natural ones. A startling omission, when one considers the sheer weight of regulation that governs our food supply chain.

For its own purposes, the food industry divides colours into two broad categories. Firstly, there are 'chemically synthesised colours'. This category includes two further sub-classes: artificial (fake) colours, and 'synthesised colours', sometimes known as 'nature identical', which are chemically identical to natural pigments, but do not come from them. Secondly, there are 'natural' colours derived from natural sources.

Confused yet? For those not initiated into the language of food manufacture, the division between thoroughly fake colours and those that have some connection, however faint, with a natural substance, is about as clear-cut as an indistinct rainbow seen from afar through rain. 'There is no clear definition of what constitutes a natural food colorant', one flavour company explains, so it is 'at the discretion of the food technologist and company developing the food product'.

In search of clarity, any food manufacturer can consult the guidelines drawn up by the Natural Food Colourings Association. It states the common-sense principle that to be described as such, a colouring must come from a pigment that occurs in nature – from plants, vegetables, flowers, algae, and so on. Fair enough. But then it goes on to say that the starting colour material can then be processed in three different ways: traditional/appropriate physical processing; traditional/appropriate physical and chemical processing; chemical synthesis.

The unthreatening word 'traditional' has a nice, low-tech ring to it, but bear in mind that in the world of food manufacturing, it is generally taken to mean any practice that has been going on for 30 years. So anyone who isn't a food technologist, or chemist, might be surprised by what the food colouring industry means by the term:

> A 'traditional process' ... includes, but is not limited to, grinding, cutting, maceration, solvent extraction, microbiological fermentation processes, heating, cooling and freezing, drying, filtration, distillation, rectification and others. A traditional process is often, but not necessarily, a physical process and can or cannot involve chemical reactions which are usually, but not always, unavoidable and unintentional.

If that sounds like stretching the meaning of the term somewhat, try 'physical':

> An 'appropriate physical process' ... includes, but is not limited to, absorption/adsorption, chromatography, ion-exchange, electrophoresis, ultrasonic treatment, centrifugation, (reverse) osmosis, crystallisation, precipitation, lyophilisation, enzymatic processes and others.

And when we come to 'chemical synthesis', we enter even deeper into a dark labyrinth of complication, from which only the professional biochemist, or chemical engineer, will emerge:

> The term 'appropriate chemical process' comprises intentionally triggered simple chemical reactions such as acidification/basification, hydrolysis, salt formation, ester cleavage, chelate formation, cis/trans- and other isomerisations.

If your head is reeling and you're thinking 'Stop, no more!', have one last attempt at getting your head around this masterfully opaque clarification:

> Depending on the concrete process, an 'appropriate chemical process' may be considered a 'traditional process' as defined above.

So, in practical terms more of us can actually understand, how are 'natural' colours actually made? Let's consider the example of the dark red viscous liquid known as paprika extract E160c. The pigment is indeed extracted from a natural source – ground up dried red peppers – but in a wholly chemical process that uses any of the following solvents (substances which dissolve it): methanol, ethanol, acetone, hexane, dichloromethane, ethyl acetate and propan-2-ol. The finished colour can, by law, contain traces of these solvents. It can also contain heavy metals – arsenic, lead, mercury and cadmium – left over from this extraction process. Of course, levels of these contaminants must be within 'safe limits', but these limits are set by food regulators who have never seriously investigated the potential cocktail effect of such substances on regular consumers of processed food.

This exceedingly inclusive interpretation of the word natural enables colour companies to create a dazzling kaleidoscope of shades – and we're not talking discreetly tasteful Farrow & Ball here. The websites and marketing materials of colouring companies are a riot of throbbing, glowing colorants – magenta from sweet potato, indigo blue from gardenia, emerald green from chlorophyllin, scarlet from elderberry, lemon yellow from safflower, orange from lutein, crimson from beetroot, royal blue from anthocyanins, slate-grey from black sesame, white from titanium, and hundreds more. Their colours, neatly grouped by general shade category, are as comprehensive as a Dulux colour chart, and even more vivid. Mind you, it would be wrong to suggest that they offer no subtlety. As the Roha colour company warns:

> Too much color can make products look too bright and unrefined in the consumers' mind. Color should be added, keeping in mind the cultural values of the sales zone and the customers' psyche.

In other words, the braying colours of a Thomas the Tank Engine birthday cake won't go down well in a chic patisserie selling macaroons in demure sugared almond shades.

Supposing you're looking for a yellow. Sensient, another colour company, can come up with several sophisticated options: 'From the greenish yellow chartreuse of your lime yoghurt to the sweet leaf vanilla fudge of your ice cream, you will find the right Sensient shade of yellow giving the desired appearance to your product.'

The selection of 'natural' colourings is so extensive, in fact, that it is potentially overwhelming. Sensient encourages manufacturers who want to brighten up their lacklustre products to dip into its 'colour book' to choose hues that will 'bring products to life'. One example is margarine-type spread, which has added yellows and oranges to change its unedifying grey appearance into an appealing primrose. 'Colour is powerful', Sensient points out. 'It can fool our taste perception producing taste differences and differentiations which do not exist.' And let's face it, margarine needs all the help it can get.

Another flavouring company, Hawkins Watts, presents food manufacturers with a full Pantone colour matching chart 'to assist your colour selection and specification process'. Food manufacturers also use its 'colour selector', a tool that helps them track down the right shade for their products. First they choose a colour range from a list, such as purple or orange, and then state whether they are looking for an artificial one. To that they must indicate what temperature the food will be processed at – high (over 100°C), medium or low – and confirm the length of time the colour must remain stable in light, choosing an option such as 'more than six months'. Finally, they must select the acidity level of the product in question, and whether or not it contains sulphur, because these factors have a further chemical effect on certain colours. For example, the yellow colouring curcumin can take on a green tint in foods with low acidity. That done, the company will recommend a shade to suit. Diana, yet another supplier of food colourings, has a 'Colour Impact Configurator' that allows manufacturers to specify with some precision the colour, shade and intensity they require.

Once food manufacturers have established the right colour for their product, they have a choice of formats. It could come as a liquid or paste mixed up in glycerine, sugar syrup, castor oil, vegetable oil, gum arabic, or even propylene glycol, the latter best known for its antifreeze potential. It can be supplied in a water-insoluble form as an aluminium 'lake', made by reacting aluminium sulfate or chloride with sodium carbonate/bicarbonate or ammonia. Although these lakes are then filtered, washed with water and dried, small traces of unreacted aluminium oxide are allowed in the final product, along with sulfates, arsenic and lead, provided they don't exceed certain limits. There are special colour forms for every use. The confectionery industry is keen on 'speed lakes', or lakes that are already dispersed in sugar syrup. Chocolatiers achieve a pearlescent effect by using colours from minerals (silica, mica) mixed in with lakes or fats. Processed meat companies like filmy coloured coatings that stick to the meat and give it a finished look. One type of caramel, for instance, will give a 'mottled black color on the surface of roast beef or Black Forest ham', while another will produce 'a uniform golden to brown coating on surface of poultry products that gives the look of oven roast turkey'. Some manufacturers use 'dyes' blended with sugars and cheap starches, such as lactose, corn starch and maltodextrin. Sometimes the colours are microencapsulated, that is, encased in vegetable fat, carbohydrates, gum or protein, inside beadlets to control their release and ensure that the shade spreads evenly through the food or beverage without leaving any tell-tale specks. Colours also come in bespoke mixtures that include a clouding agent. These 'cloudifiers', usually oil mixed with gum, lend a translucent effect. Cloudy colours are used particularly by drinks manufacturers because they help give consumers the impression that their products contain more real fruit juice pulp than they actually do. As one industry manual explains:

> A soft drink with low natural juice content may require a clouding agent to boost the turbidity [haziness] in order for it to resemble the cloudy natural juice of the fruit it is named after.

The technology of natural colours is advanced and elaborate, allowing food manufacturers plenty of scope for artful creativity in shaping our perceptions of what we eat and drink. Their interpretation of 'natural' does not reflect most consumers' understanding of, or hopes for, that term, yet this hasn't stopped food manufacturers taking advantage of the move away from artificial colours for marketing purposes. Our supermarkets are full of products plastered with prominent 'no artificial colours', 'free from' logos and tick lists, most prominently on food for infants and children. Such labels instantly put a ring of virtue around a product, and lull us into thinking that there's no need to look in more forensic detail at the ingredients listing.

Cashing in on 'natural' has its limits though. Despite the generally laissez-faire regulation of food colourings, the hard fact for food manufacturers is that European law does at least insist that whether artificial or 'natural', any added food colouring must be labelled as such. Along with the designation 'colour', manufacturers can choose to declare it either by name or E number. They have some discretion about how they do that. They can use the name, say lutein, along with the explanatory words 'natural food colour', or they can list this yellow colour by its E (additive) number, E161b. But there's no getting around the requirement that any added colour must be declared, however small and hard to read, in the ingredients listing on the back of the product. And when observant shoppers spot that, it makes them wonder about the breezy 'free from' claims on the front of the pack.

Anticipating that public suspicion of food colourings was bound to grow, the processed food industry, always a step ahead, has in recent years come up with a sparkling new concept: 'colouring foods'. The sales pitch here is that instead of using added colourings as we know them, either artificial or natural, bright pigments extracted from foods such as beetroot, spinach and paprika, are being used.

On first sight, colouring foods are an engaging proposition, not least because vegetable and plant names always bestow a highly desirable botanical probity on a product. But are colouring foods really as benign as they might seem? While it would be wrong to imply that food manufacturers are simply engaged in a cynical rebadging exercise, the truth is there is no bright blue sea, nor clear red line, between 'natural colours' and 'colouring foods'. As the FSA diplomatically puts it: 'Both industry and regulators consider there is a difficult legislative boundary between a food colour additive and a colouring food.'

In recent years, companies have largely done their own thing, developing colouring foods with enthusiasm, and using terms such as beetroot extract, roasted barley malt extract and carrot concentrate to describe them. To most consumers this sounds progressive, even medicinally beneficial, and of course it allows manufacturers more scope for cleaner labels with prominent 'no nasties'-type claims. From a commercial point of view, colourful food extracts have the additional benefit of being easier to bring to market. Under European law, food colourings, both artificial and 'natural', require pre-marketing approval and safety assessment. 'Colouring foods', on the other hand, don't, because they are classed as ingredients, not additives. So, a further bonus, they don't need to be labelled with those pesky E numbers either.

In 2014, the European Commission belatedly issued guidance designed to clarify matters: as long as a substance has not been selectively extracted from a natural food it can be marketed as a 'colouring food'. But in yet another demonstration of the blurry, watercolour language of food colours, 'selective extraction' is an obligingly loose term. It 'leaves some room for preparations obtained from foods using a process of physical and/or chemical extraction which may be interpreted as not being selectively extracted', and 'extraction can range from simple extraction, to degrees of selective extraction'. The practical test of whether something has been selectively extracted or not comes down to two factors – enrichment and purity – both of which involve ratio calculations. Just as when accountants prepare complicated tax returns, it is a matter of interpretation. One company's carrot root extract might possibly qualify as a 'colouring food' while another company's does not.

And some of the ingredients used as colouring foods might not be to everyone's taste. For instance, the Belgian company Veos markets red blood cells for colouring meat:

> The stabilised red cells are used as a natural colouring agent, without E-number as a colorant! This protein is perfect to improve the colour of meat products and to increase the meat perception. After cooking hams for instance, a nice homogeneous meat colour will be reached, even when working with PSE meat.

PSE, by the way, stands for pale soft exudative. PSE meat has an abnormal colour, and looks dry. The UN's Food and Agriculture Organization explains why this happens:

> PSE in pigs is caused by severe, short-term stress just prior to slaughter, for example during off-loading, handling, holding in pens and stunning. Here the animal is subjected to severe anxiety and fright caused by manhandling, fighting in the pens and bad stunning techniques. All this may result in biochemical processes in the muscle, in particular, in rapid breakdown of muscle glycogen and the meat becoming very pale with pronounced acidity and poor flavour.

So poor quality meat, from stressed-out animals, turns out a nice healthy-looking pink when coloured pink with blood cells. Mmm, nice.

The bottom line here is that the boundary between 'natural colourings' and 'colouring foods' is about as clear as mud, and exists only in the form of meek industry guidance, not meticulously defined law.

In fact, the guidance notes come with this puzzling disclaimer: 'These guidance notes do not represent the official position of the Commission and they do not intend to produce legally binding effects.' Which makes you wonder about the point of the whole exercise. Cynicism only grows when you know that these guidance notes were 'elaborated by Commission services after consultation with the Member States' experts on food additives and the relevant stakeholders'. Considering that the aforementioned 'member states' experts' are frequently chemical industry scientists who have captured influential positions on government committees, and 'relevant stakeholders' is code for companies active in the food additive business, it's hard not to draw the conclusion that the colouring industry is writing its own lurid rules.

10

Watery

Before I began investigating them for this book, ready-to-eat meats were a bit of a mystery to me, just because they were so different in form, texture and taste from any meats I have ever cooked at home. The first thing that struck me as strange was that they shared a certain sheen; it reminds me of the effect you get when petrol and water mix accidentally on the paving of a rainy petrol station forecourt. Whenever I cook meat, once the initial sheen of heat has gone, it looks matt, rather than shiny, with a variation in colour: some parts are pink, others much darker. Texture was a further puzzler. No meat cooked at home by me, or anyone else I know for that matter, has the slippery humidity and 'bounce' that is a hallmark of processed, cooked meats. At the firm end of the spectrum lie products with a Spam-like firmness, things like tinned ham, hot dogs, luncheon meat and garlic sausage. In the middle ground, there are those that have a bit of a wobble, offering an elastic resistance in the mouth. Think of the chicken discs that parents are encouraged to slip into their children's lunch-box. At the softer end, you get those floppy yet still cohesive slices of ham with the clamminess of a limp, damp hand-shake; the sort that turns up in your workplace cafeteria sandwich, or on top of your pizza. And then there was the conundrum of the shape. No home-boiled ham or turkey I ever came across carved obligingly into identical slices of the same dimensions.

As I soon discovered, the distinctive characteristics of these ready-cooked meats are a testament to the boundless creativity, food engineering skill and sheer thrift of meat processors. Their art consists of taking a sow's ear (often literally), and turning it into a silk purse. They do this by reconfiguring meat and fish in an infinitely more profitable way, through the addition of water. Lots of it. Why? Water is cheap; meat and seafood are expensive. The economic logic of such 'cost engineering', as it is known in food manufacturing, is obvious. Why sell meat when you can sell added water?

That said, getting meat to absorb liquid isn't an easy task; in fact it's contrary to the laws of nature. When an animal or fish dies, its muscles naturally contract (rigor mortis) and expel moisture. In the natural world, meat and fish get drier as they age, not wetter, and when we cook them, they dry out further. Nevertheless, meat manufacturers get round that technical challenge by mixing together tap water with a variety of substances, some classed as ingredients, some as processing aids, some as food additives, to make a soaking solution, referred to in the trade as 'brine'. The substances added to the water vary in nature and composition, but they all have one thing in common: they act as binders, encouraging the meat or fish to do something it would not otherwise do: soak up and retain water.

So what tools for this purpose do meat manufacturers have at their disposal? For starters, there's transglutaminase, an enzyme. Its use is now widespread in meat processing. One company that markets it to meat manufacturers explains to its prospective customers that it works by 'catalyzing reactions in the formation of covalent bonds between a carboxylamide group of the lateral chain on a glutamine residue and the amino group of the lateral chain of a lysine'. Pardon me? Try understanding that little lot if you aren't a biochemist. But food manufacturers can ignore all that and cut to the chase. Transglutaminase creates strong bonds between proteins, the company says, and thus 'transforms worthless cuts of meat or fish without commercial value into standardised portions with a high added value'. Now we're talking a language that everyone can understand.

No wonder transglutaminase is known in the trade as 'meat glue'. It gets bits of meat or fish to stick together that wouldn't otherwise do so. It gives manufacturers the properties they deem essential – juicy firmness, elasticity, viscosity and 'thermo-stability' (the meat retains these other qualities when heated), and so 'facilitates the addition of water'.

Transglutaminase has another benefit for meat processors: it reduces the traditional drying and maturing time needed for cured meats, such as salami, by up to 40 per cent. So it provides a nifty short cut for manufacturers of all types of charcuterie products sold on deli counters up and down the land. For instance, one Romanian company, Supremia, produces a transglutaminase product blended with animal protein and vitamin B9:

> Salami Dry Express B9 decreases ripening time by up to 20 per cent, creates a more homogenous and appealing colour in less time, offers improved casing peeling and enhanced sausage aroma. Improved slicing properties reduce wastage

> by up to five per cent, while shorter processing and storage times also provide financial advantages. A special ripening room [for maturing the salami] is not needed.

Conveniently for manufacturers the European Commission, doubtless under pressure from those same manufacturers, has classified transglutaminase as a processing aid rather than an ingredient, because 'the end-product production process – normally the application of heat – inactivates enzymes or depletes the substrates, meaning that transglutaminase is not present in the final product'. So, with a little bit of semantic manipulation, transglutaminase is 'clean label' and it doesn't have to be listed on the packaging. This means that irrespective of whether or not you shop for cooked meat and charcuterie in high- or low-end shops, there is no way you will ever know if it was made with the aid of transglutaminase. Equally, simply by reading the label, you won't have a clue whether your salami or ham was cured the patient, traditional way, or speeded up by the use of this enzyme. However posh and artisan some cured meats might appear, in this respect their pedigree is a little hazy.

Phosphates are another useful class of chemicals in the meat processor's batterie de cuisine. Derived from phosphoric acid, phosphates 'raise the pH (of meat) and work with salt to increase the ionic strength, which favours protein solubilisation and water absorption'. Or, in other words, phosphates make protein soluble so that it develops a natural tackiness that will bind meat or fish pieces with water. Maybe you have tried to fry bacon, only to find that it exudes a cloudy white liquid that prevents it crisping? That's undissolved phosphate and added water seeping out. Manufacturers have to be careful to get the dosage of phosphate just right, because fat and phosphate combine to make soap, and some people with keen taste buds will pick up a soapy taste in phosphate-swollen meat. Nothing that a bit of extra salt, sugar and flavouring can't disguise, mind you.

Phosphates are pretty essential kit for manufacturing boneless hams, chicken and turkey roll, bacon and charcuterie, but they are also used extensively in seafood processing. The delicate nature of seafood proteins causes them to denature far more rapidly than those of meat and poultry, and the Omega-3 fats in fish and shellfish are also highly prone to oxidation, which causes them to discolour as they age, first to yellow, then to brown, and finally blue. And who wants to eat old, stinky, matt-looking seafood when, as any good fishmonger will tell you, fresh fish should have a natural sparkle? Phosphates allow processors to extend the shelf life of seafood by preventing the protein degrading and so developing a telltale rancid flavour and changed colour.

By dipping fish fillets in a solution of phosphates and water, seafood processors create a surface coating of dissolved proteins on the fillets, which then forms a protein glue when frozen. Result? As one phosphate company coyly puts it, the fillets will 'retain natural juices for a longer period of time', and of course, with all the water now soaked into them, the fish will weigh much more than it did to start with.

While phosphate treatment makes a perceptible difference to the texture of meat, in shellfish the effect is particularly remarkable. A natural scallop, sold 'dry', that is not treated with phosphates, will be relatively small, with a fresh marine sweetness to it, and a pleasingly springy texture. The same scallop, sold 'wet', that is treated with phosphates, will look about twice the size, taste of next to nothing, and have a jellied consistency. When the FSA tested fresh raw scallops, it found that nearly half of samples tested contained more than 10 per cent added water, and some samples had as much as 54 per cent.

Still, scallops pumped up with phosphates and water are extremely attractive to restaurateurs and chefs who want to cut their ingredient costs. The odd customer might notice that the bivalves were disappointing to eat and vaguely wonder why, but many more will tuck into them, feeling that they are getting a generous portion for the price.

Phosphates are also used as a 'processing aid' for prawn shelling. They 'solubilise' the collagen protein that attaches the prawn to its shell so that the prawns exude less liquid when they are defrosted, yet the word phosphate does not have to appear on the label. Phosphates also play a vital role in the manufacture of mass-produced scampi, which are scraps of prawn 'reformed' to look like whole prawn tail, and surimi, the imitation crabmeat. Surimi is made by repeatedly washing a mulch of white fish, then adding a blend of phosphates, sweeteners such as sucrose and sorbitol, pink colouring and artificial crab flavouring. Without the last ingredient, by the time it goes through the manufacturing process, surimi would have no flavour whatsoever. You may not be aware of ever eating surimi, but it often turns up in the middle of sushi rolls. Masked by wasabi (pungent horseradish) and salty soy sauce, it supplies texture and colour, and its lack of flavour goes by unnoticed.

Hydrocolloids, a group of gummy sweet starches, are another set of ingredients that bind flesh to water. In this group come carrageenan and agar (derived from seaweed), gum acacia and locust bean (from trees), guar gum, inulin, cellulose and konjac (from plants), xanthan (made by fermenting corn sugar with a bacterium), and pectin (from fruits). Hydrocolloids are used extensively in food processing, for making everything from ice cream and milk shake through to sauces and gravies. Just a small amount added to a recipe – only 1, or even 0.5 per cent – will make any liquid ingredient thicker and more viscous, and bind those that would otherwise split, 'shear' and separate out. A dash of xanthan gum, for instance, will stabilise the oil, water and vinegar emulsion in an off-the-shelf salad dressing.

In the meat manufacturing business, hydrocolloids help do the all-important job of uniting bits of boned meat and water in a highly lucrative, sticky embrace. According to one company that supplies carrageenan, meat processors who use this gum can improve the 'yield' or weight of their products by as much as 100 per cent. Carrageenan is supplied to the trade in three different forms – kappa, iota and lambda – depending on how jellied a 'mouthfeel' is required. Hydrocolloids appeal to retailers too. Thanks to their binding properties, meat products that contain them cut very cleanly. Nice neat slices; no wastage; tidy profit margins.

Hydrocolloids and phosphates are hardly cutting edge, and now many meat manufacturers prefer to substitute, or include in the brine formulation, a group of highly refined starchy fibres and flours with a high water-holding capacity, extracted from sources as diverse as wheat, soya, peas, bamboo, rice, potatoes and citrus. Commonly used in products such as sausages, pâtés, meatballs and meat pie fillings, the sales pitch for these flours and fibres is that they 'tightly bind added water in processed meat products to improve yields and profits'. Their 'sponge effect' makes a big contribution to the weight of raw, boned poultry meat. One company with a buoyant business in the field claims that adding just half a kilo to 100 litres of brine 'significantly reduces storage drip'. Plainly put, if your chicken supremes have had some starchy fibre added to their brine, they will hold added water and form less of a puddle when they defrost.

Starchy fibres of this type are used to firm up, or, as the industry prefers to put it, 'retexturise' chicken products, such as Kievs and nuggets, that have been 'restructured'. In 'emulsion' products, where meat is processed until it forms a slurry, a slightly more substantial dosage of starchy fibre will provide the much firmer consistency and bouncy 'snap' that allows a frankfurter or knackwurst to break cleanly in two.

The makers of one such starchy fibre product, Swelite®, based on yellow peas, explain its function. The evocatively named Swelite® 'improves the processability, stability, texture and yield of the final product'. Moreover, 'it can replace 50 to 100% of a protein source while improving juiciness'. In other words, Swelite® allows meat processors to radically reduce the amount of meat needed in their recipe. Not for nothing is 'making the most of meat' the marketing slogan for Swelite®.

The makers of another starch-based instant texturiser, Ultra Create, spell out its usefulness to manufacturers and caterers: 'Ultra Create instant texturiser can help food processors and foodservice establishments quickly create delicious soups, sauces, gravies and dry mixes with minimal effort and energy'. Products made with this texturiser are 'freeze/thaw stable, allowing foodservice establishments to prepare formulations in advance without concern about them breaking down or gelling during processing or reheating', it explains. Note the 'minimal effort and energy' bit: that's what food processing is all about.

Soya protein is another useful 'meat extender' for manufacturers. It comes in the ready-to-use forms of flour, concentrate or protein isolate. This processed soya protein is typically extracted by washing soya flour in acid, in aluminium tanks, introducing the possibility that this heavy metal, which is known to be bad for the brain and the nervous system, can leach into the product. The chemical solvent, hexane – a component in glue and cement – is also used in the soya protein extraction process. Hexane is known to poison the nervous system, although the soya industry insists that no hexane residues find their way into the finished product.

But why would manufacturers use such a controversial ingredient? Soya is the plant food that comes closest to having the texture of meat, and it has a prodigious ability to absorb water and fat. So, according to the UN's Food and Agriculture Organization, it can be used to replace as much as 30 per cent of the meat in products such as sausages, pie fillings, meat sauces, ready meals and meatballs. And because soya proteins are considerably cheaper than meat, manufacturers have a strong financial reason to do so.

Some manufacturers still use gelatine, a highly refined form of collagen, the protein found in animal tendons, ligaments and skin. Collagen is sticky stuff; the word comes from the ancient Greek 'kolla', meaning glue. It forms 'stiff fibres of tremendous tensile strength' and 'loosely woven fibres, permitting expansion in all directions'. Gelatine is obtained from animal carcasses after all their meat has been removed in the abattoir, in a chemical process that uses an acid or alkali solution, or enzymes, and water, to break down the raw material. If gelatine is used in a meat product, it has to be listed as an ingredient on the label, and these days it is beginning to look a bit last century. In recent years, meat manufacturers have begun to use a newer, 'clean label', more 'functional' form of collagen protein powder with a slightly different chemical structure, obtained in a chemical process where the proteins are extracted from the animal by-products using mechanical and heat treatment. Functional proteins of this type are rising stars in the contemporary meat processing firmament. In the language of food manufacturing, they guarantee improved 'sliceability', firmness and cohesiveness, producing that juicy, slightly resistant 'mouthfeel' that we associate with processed meats, and reduce 'purge' (the seepage of watery liquid into the product pack) by acting as a barrier to water loss. As one supplier of chemicals to food manufacturers puts it: 'Proteins, thanks to their multi functionalities like solubility, viscosity, water binding, emulsifying, gelation, cohesion, foaming and elasticity, bring a specific impact to food systems.'

Manufacturers have various methods for adding proteins to their products. In the case of fish fillets, these can be injected with a solution of fish protein hydrolysate (FPH) or homogenised fish proteins (HFP). Alternatively, these substances can be included in a brine. If you're talking sausages or meatballs, then the protein powder can be added directly to the meat mix along with the corresponding amount of water to produce a springy consistency. Alternatively, the powder can be whisked with water until it forms a cloudy gel, which then sets to form a very firm jelly with the pliant 'give' of a stress ball. This substance, which looks white, beige or brown, depending on whether pig, cow or poultry collagen has been used, can then be canned, pasteurised and stored at room temperature until it is needed, ready for mixing into a range of 'meat applications', everything from burgers and chicken supremes to meat fillings and salami. Manufacturers also use a sprinkling of collagen powder to add heft, and a glossy thickness, to gravies and ready meals, such as a cottage pie or roast beef dinner.

Protein powders are extremely attractive to meat processors for two reasons. Firstly, they allow for a more 'natural' label. The only ingredient listing needed will be 'beef protein', 'poultry protein' or 'pork protein', which is unlikely to cause alarm. We all know that we need protein to build muscles, right? Secondly, when reconstituted with water, protein powders can be used as a direct substitute for a significant proportion of the meat and fat in a formulation, and so, in the words of one company, 'beef up their sales'.

Here's how the figures stack up. A manufacturer pays £1.85 a kilo for 'beef trim' (scraps of boned, frozen beef supplied ready for processing) but only £0.85 a kilo for beef protein powder. By replacing 10 per cent of the beef with protein powder and water, an industrial-size meat processing company using 200 tons of meat a week can make a significant weekly saving of £20,000. And with supermarkets exerting constant pressure on suppliers to keep their prices unfeasibly low, this is precisely the sort of cost adjustment that allows manufacturers to make some money. As one protein company puts it: 'Functional proteins allow you to replace more expensive ingredients in your application, thereby reducing cost while increasing yield.'

Food manufacturers can also choose functional proteins derived from blood, for instance plasma. The Belgian company, Veos, explains:

> Plasma proteins have an enormous water binding capacity. At temperatures above 65°C, the albumin proteins form a 3-dimensional network which becomes a strong and heat-stable gel. This gel-forming property, as well as the high solubility in brines, makes the protein-enriching product well suitable for injection in cooked hams [sic]. Plasma is also used in cuttered and ground meat products where a strong 'meat bite' is needed, especially when the meat product is eaten warm like frankfurters.

Alternatively, in a deli counter pâté perhaps, globin might be more suitable:

> The allergen-free protein is an excellent emulsifier as it stabilises the water/fat/protein matrix [mix] in cuttered and ground meat products. By consequence, it prevents fat and water separation before, during and after cooking. In preparation of warm emulsions (like pâté, liver sausage) one part of globin stabilises 20 parts of hot water and 20 parts of hot fat. For emulsified products where we use cold raw materials, 1 part of globin easily binds 7 parts of fat and ice.

Like collagen, a dash of added blood products does wonders for a manufacturer's profit margins. They're easy to get hold of too, 'sold through a worldwide sales network in over 70 countries on six continents'.

Transglutaminase, phosphates, hydrocolloids, starchy fibres, soya, gelatine, protein powders – meat processors can deploy a catholic selection of ingredients and processing aids to add water to meat. Many choose a belt and braces approach, using several of them at a time, along with other additives.

Here are two typical formulations:

A recipe for hot dogs
Ingredients:
Fatty meat (58%)
Meat with tendons (7.2%)
Bloodied cuts (actual wording) (7.2%)
Water (21.4%)
Functional premix (phosphate, monosodium glutamate [MSG], antioxidant, sodium citrate, colour) (1%)
Wheat fibre (1%)
Starch (2%)
Spice mix (0.6%)
Nitrite salt – a preservative (1.6%)

A recipe for bacon brine
Ingredients:
Water (83.38%)
Carrageenan (1.25%)
Sodium nitrite – a preservative (0.10%)
Sodium erythorbate – a preservative (0.50%)
Dextrose – a sugar (1.50%)
Sodium citrate – an antioxidant and acidity regulator (0.75%)
Salt (9%)
Phosphates (1.50%)

Collagen protein (2.00%)
Xanthan gum (0.02%)

The business of adding water to meat is relatively easy when you're talking about emulsified products, such as hot dogs and mortadella, or 'comminuted' products, like burgers, sausages and meatballs, because the meat is already minced up or pulverised, the cells have been broken down and are more absorbent. But special equipment is needed to encourage more intact cuts, hams or chicken breast for instance, to soak it up; 'static absorption', as it's known in the meat business, just won't do the trick.

So manufacturers can 'tumble' the meat along with the brine in a vacuum machine that looks a bit like a sealed version of a drum concrete mixer. As the tumbler drum rotates, steel paddles inside it slowly move the meat pieces to create a mechanical massaging effect, which helps it absorb the watery solution and free protein from the meat tissue. Once heat treated or cooked, usually in plastic bags in steam or water baths, this semi-liquid protein, along with added chemicals, binds the meat pieces firmly together, making it look like one intact joint.

A brine injector machine is another useful bit of kit. Meats are fed into it on a moving belt and injected repeatedly with the brine using several rows of needles that puncture the flesh, creating tiny cavities, and transporting the solution deep into the cells of the meat, effectively turning it into a sponge. Needle brine injectors are extensively used for processing boned bacon, ham and chicken breast, but not for whole birds, because the needles would puncture the skin and leave black marks. However, poultry processors can instead use injectors fitted with high-pressure nozzles to 'inject' the brine, so that the meat can pick up more water. The makers of one such machine claim that it can inject 12,000 chickens an hour, 'without the hassle of blisters'.

Whether they have been dipped, tumbled or injected, or had a sack load of binders added directly into the mix, many of the cured and ready-cooked meats we eat, however substantial they might feel, are awash with water, and when we buy them, we are paying through the nose for water laced with chemicals. In 2013, when the *Guardian* revealed that major supermarkets were selling, perfectly legally, frozen chicken breasts with 18 per cent added water, the newspaper calculated that consumers who bought them would be paying about 65 pence a kilo for water. When the *Daily Mail* carried out its own investigation subsequently, it concluded that the figure was actually much higher, £1.54 a kilo to be precise.

In the processed meat trade, the term 'liquid lunch' takes on a whole new meaning.

11

Starchy

If you're a dedicated home cook, you might have a packet of cornflour or arrowroot at the back of a cupboard – to make custard perhaps, or thicken a fruit sauce – but starch is not a core grocery item for most people. And why would it be? Starch is an uninspiring ingredient. This common carbohydrate derived from plant foods such as corn, wheat, potato, cassava and rice, is white, powdery, tasteless and odourless. In itself, it is a non-event, a heap of nothingness, about as exciting to eat as wallpaper paste; indeed, it is used for precisely that purpose.

In food manufacturing, however, starch is essential kit, by far the most commonly used item in the food manufacturer's box of tricks, as one authority explains: 'Since their development in the 1940s, modified food starches have become a vital part of the food industry. Practically every category of food utilises the functional properties of starch to impart some important aspect of the final product.'

It's no exaggeration to say that the modern processed food industry is predicated on the stuff. This is why, when you turn to the ingredients listings on the massed ranks of manufactured foods, the word starch turns up with regularity, sometimes prefixed by a source, say, potato starch, or more often by the enigmatic word 'modified'.

Although it is an omnipresent ingredient in many foods we regularly eat, few of us understand the role that starch plays in specific products; and because it is so ubiquitous, only the most wary of us question its use, not least because alongside all those ingredients and additives with long science lab names, starch sounds like the very least of our problems.

Food manufacturers, on the other hand, are fully aware of the myriad uses and applications for this anonymous commodity. Starch acts as a muse for the modern food industry, a biddable, versatile, obliging substance that inspires a never-ending flow of creativity. Although it is utterly lacking in any food personality of its own, the very neutrality of nondescript starch makes everything feasible. Think of it as a facilitator, an ingredient that generates a boundless range of technical possibilities.

Added starch makes puffed potato snacks and breakfast cereals crisp and expansive, it makes your tortilla chip crunchier, and your crisps crispier. It lends smoothness and creaminess to processed cheese. It extends the shelf life of yogurt, gels fruit and cream fillings, adds fibre to bread, replaces eggs, makes batter more clingy, adds porosity to crackers, and airiness to cakes. In tumbled, injected and emulsified meats, such as sausages and ham, it can mimic fat, so acting as a 'meat extender'. Starch seals in moist glazes and marinades and acts as a carrier for flavourings and colourings. Thanks to starch, you can transport your mousse dessert upside down and it will emerge unruffled. It stops your orange juice from separating and makes it cloudy. Starch binds the water in mayonnaise, margarine, ketchup and salad dressings, toughens up dough for the onslaught of factory baking, and adds viscous heft to bouillons and gravies. It stiffens canned foods – soups, pulses, vegetables – and makes ready meals more resilient to the temperature challenges posed by chilling, freezing, transportation, reheating, and the general stress and elevated temperatures of factory production. Starch provides 'freeze/thaw stability', prevents freezer 'burn' (damage to food from freezing) and gives food more 'microwave tolerance'. Last but not least, it can create a texture. Whatever consistency is needed – crisp, crunchy, melting, creamy, succulent, gummy, mouth filling, elastic, smooth, shreddable, jellied, stringy, cuttable, short, smooth, cohesive or chewy – multi-tasking starch can deliver it.

Food manufacturers love starch for its 'functionality'. Not only does starch make it practical to create a long list of manufactured food and drink products that would otherwise be totally unfeasible, starch is not fazed by the tough requirements of industrial food production. Its virtues for manufacturers are numerous, and according to one authority they include 'adhesion, antistaling, binding, clouding, dusting, emulsion stabilisation, encapsulation, flowing aid, foam strengthening, gelling, glazing, moisture retention, molding, shaping, stabilising and thickening'. Starch truly is a miraculous ingredient that fulfils a whole catalogue of manufacturing needs.

But how can one boring, anodyne ingredient do so much? After all, starch in the form that ordinary people know it, such as cornflour and arrowroot, can only perform a fraction of the tasks mentioned above. As you might have guessed, the starches available to food manufacturers are rather remote relatives of those we might use at home. They have been altered in various ways to endow them with properties they lack in any of their recognised household forms. As one group of researchers puts it: 'Food manufacturers generally prefer starches with better behavioral characteristics than those provided by native [natural] starches.' Natural starches, you see, are badly behaved, dysfunctional starches that can only ever find their true potential through the improving hand of food technology.

Modified starch, the most familiar of these 'improved', more 'functional' starches, has clocked up decades of steadfast services to industrial food manufacture. This type of starch can be made using various techniques to change (modify) its characteristics. These include breaking it down with acids, bleaching it, converting it with enzymes, pre-gelatinising it by heating and drying it so that it forms a gel in cold water, oxidising it, cross-linking it with fats, converting it into esters or ethers, and bonding it with phosphates. Starch can also be browned using dry heat (dextrinisation) to turn it into 'starch sugars', such as maltodextrin. Put it this way, modified starch is definitely not something you could cook up in any home kitchen.

There are many types of modified starch, each with unique properties and functions, a case of horses for courses. The starch in canned soups, for example, is often bonded with phosphates, which allows it to absorb more water yet stop any separation in the liquid. To prevent tomato sauce spilling off a factory pizza during baking, a modified starch treated with a chlorine solution is often added to the topping.

In Europe, modified starches are considered as food additives, and must carry an E number. These days, because the prefix 'modified' tends to ring the wrong bell with consumers, starch companies are developing a new tier of more functional 'clean label' starches that can lose the label-polluting M-word and E number, and be replaced with more consumer-friendly 'soluble fibre', 'starch' or 'dextrin' tags.

These new wave starches are presented as more natural because they have not been chemically altered. Instead, only physical and mechanical techniques such as heat, extrusion, drum drying, compression and atomisation can be used to change the particle size and structure. Because these newer functional starches are branded and trademarked, the companies that produce them need only volunteer minimal information about how they are made because the method becomes their intellectual property (trade secret). Marketed as speciality starches targeted for specific uses, they have really caught on with manufacturers. As one academic explains, 'specialty starches continue to outpace unmodified starches in the processed food industry because of their ruggedness and ability to withstand severe process conditions'.

It's easy to see why food manufacturers take such a keen interest in starch, both old-timer and new guard. Whether it comes from corn, wheat, cassava, peas or potato, starch is wonderfully cheap and abundant because it is made from commodity cereals and cash crops that are much less expensive than other categories of food. Therein lies the appeal of starch. It provides a reliable, inexpensive bulk to pad out pricier ingredients, which makes for cost-effective ingredient replacement, as this starch company tells food manufacturers:

> Like you, we're committed to keeping costs low. Our business is built on successfully replacing expensive ingredients with more cost-effective alternatives, helping you withstand

> price fluctuations. Whether replicating expensive texture systems or substituting costly proteins, our starches will meet all your expectations and reduce your ingredient costs. So what's the secret of creating foods that appeal to customers' concerns about cost and quality? Take a fresh look at your recipes and replace expensive ingredients with no-compromise alternatives to reduce cost, not consumer appeal. We can provide you with the tools to replicate the eating enjoyment and texture consumers look for at a fraction of the cost.

The most charitable interpretation one can put on food manufacturers' use of economical starch is that they deploy it in the best interests of the consumer, to give us what we want, at a price we can afford. With the aid of starch, manufacturers can use 'cost optimisation' to 'value engineer' their product for the benefit of price-sensitive shoppers. A worthwhile mission, surely?

Yet when you read the sales literature for starch products, a strong sense of self-interest on the part of food manufacturers emerges. Here, for instance, is how one starch company sells its starch-based fat replacer:

> [It] cleverly allows food manufacturers to remove some butter content from products and still use the label 'all butter', which highlights to consumers that the food is still a decadent product. The finish of the product would retain the same 'shortness' and buttery richness and mouth-feel as the full fat equivalent.

Hey presto, the addition of starch allows opulently labelled 'all butter' biscuits or croissants to contain less butter than they did before. Not quite what your average person might deduce from the label. The fat-replacing starch being recommended here goes by the name of Delyte, presumably a play on delight/delicious and lite/light (low fat). Or possibly the person who thought it up was thinking of delete, meaning something taken away; in this case, butter.

In food manufacturing, starch often forms the basis of a product. 'Your base starch serves as a viscosifier, which establishes your food's structure', one company explains. An example here might be a Catalan-style flan or French crème caramel, where starch replaces more expensive eggs, milk and cream. 'Once you've created the structure with your base starch, co-texturisers [another set of starches] fine-tune texture properties. They bring out the more subtle differences in texture that we experience in our mouths while eating, such as mouthcoating [creamy] and meltaway [lusciousness].'

As well as offering cheap bulk and texturising potential, starch has never been in such demand as it currently is to replace other nutrients. As health regulators have breathed ever so lightly down the neck of the processed food industry to make its products healthier, reduction of fat, sugar and salt has become a regulatory religion, one that opens new doors for starch. Products can be reformulated, bumping up quantities of starch and cutting the persona non grata ingredients, thus providing a justification for reduced fat and sugar claims on the label. Using starch, manufacturers can adjust the composition or 'matrix' of a whole host of processed foods, to recast them in a flattering nutritional light. Doing so ticks a few boxes with the public health establishment, and the sums also add up very nicely for manufacturers, as this starch company explains:

> Our specialty solutions mimic the organoleptic qualities of fat, delivering a creamy, luxurious texture and smooth, glossy appearance in better-for-you applications. We're also skilled at replacing costly tomato solids. Whether you are looking to replace oil, cream, milk solids, vegetables or egg, we can ensure premium quality and guilt-free indulgence at a competitive price.

And when it comes to starch, ingredient savings are no idle promise. A high-performance starch can replace fat at a ratio of 10:1 in dips, dressings, soups and mayonnaise for a lower calorie, lower fat label at a lower cost. Starch can stand in for 30% of the cream in a ready meal spaghetti carbonara and make redundant at least 25% of the tomato paste otherwise needed to make a credible pasta sauce. It allows manufacturers to reduce the margarine in puff pastry by a fifth. A starch developed using a 'cling optimised texture system' will even have the necessary adhesion, viscosity and suspension to replace 'up to 40% of tomato/vegetable solids in soups and sauces'.

On a factory scale, using starch makes for massive savings. As one food industry commentator observed, 'Food technologists are a creative, but miserly, crowd. They strive to deliver consumer-pleasing products while piecing together penny-saving formulas'. Unlike home cooks, food technologists think in terms not of ingredients, but 'ingredient systems'. For instance, rather than using an egg, they can come up with a configuration of ingredients and additives, which in totality will provide an egg-like effect. And in this endeavour, starch is a near-indispensable tool.

Of course, mimicry lies at the heart of modern food manufacture, a constant itch to make not a faithful version of the real thing, but something that passes for it. For food technologists and new product developers, all the fun with food comes when you take it apart, break it down into components, then reassemble it in a more lucrative, easy-to-process form.

Greek yogurt is a case in point. It is the most copied food of recent times, not least because its desirable 'spoonability' is pushing phenomenal market growth: sales grew by an impressive 67 per cent between 2008 and 2012. The spectacular sales curve of thick, rich Greek yogurt is symptomatic of growing disenchantment with dismal low-fat yogurts, a reaction to the sensory gap created by the removal of fat, the fraction of milk that naturally contains most of its taste and gives it a mouth-filling creaminess.

Sensing an opportunity, many companies want to get in on the dynamic Greek yogurt sector. As the spokesman for one dairy company notes: 'Greek and Greek-style yoghurts often command a significant price premium in store, and offer food manufacturers an excellent opportunity to increase their margins'. But they face a stumbling block. When produced in the traditional way, Greek yogurt takes a whole lot more milk to make than standard yogurt, which puts up ingredient costs. Using an authentic Greek method, you need 100 kg of milk to end up with just 40 kg of finished yogurt. You'll also require special separation equipment, and all that heroic Hellenic straining takes time. Who can be fagged? So the food industry has developed 'quick process' Greek-style yogurt that yields 100 kg of yogurt for 100 kg of milk, without having to buy equipment, or radically change factory set-up, by adding milk protein concentrate and starch. The resulting product is not authentic Greek yogurt as the Greeks understand it, but it will pass muster with many consumers, and the telling word 'style' will mainly go unremarked.

One market leading starch company, Ingredion, explains how it brought starch to the Greek yogurt arena:

> The company employed its trained expert descriptive sensory panel to evaluate nine Greek-style yogurt samples on the market, all vanilla flavored, most strained, but some formulated, and characterised each one by 14 different textural attributes.

The company first mapped the sensory attributes of Greek yogurts on the market: qualities such as 'jiggle' (how firmly the yogurt moves on the spoon), 'slipperiness' (how easily it slides over the tongue), and surface shine. It then devised an innovative starch, which it claims can give 'a similar texture and eating experience to the market leading product', yet is cheaper to produce because it uses less milk and can be made using the standard high temperature/short time non-Greek method, without any investment in new equipment. With this fabulously functional starch, Ingredion promises that yogurt manufacturers 'can get to market faster, and produce product at a lower overall cost'.

How does fast-track Greek-ish yogurt compare in taste to the genuine article? Because most such products are sold not as natural, plain yogurt, but with added flavours and sweeteners, we rarely have the opportunity to compare like for like. However, it is common knowledge in the processed food industry that starch can import unwelcome flavours. As one authority notes: 'Cereal-based starches such as corn and wheat starch are sometimes considered to have off-notes described as 'cardboard' or 'cereal-like'. Fortunately for manufacturers, because most processed foods are multiple ingredient formulations, they can make sure that off-tastes are routinely drowned out by other attention-grabbing flavours.

One thing is certain: the addition of starch reduces flavour in food. This is not just because it is used as a substitute for flavourful ingredients – eggs, meat, cheese, butter and so on – either. The hard fact is that starch brings absolutely nothing desirable to the table except texture, so eating food bulked up with added starch is the taste equivalent of listening to a symphony orchestra through a heavy fire door. Flavours become indistinct and ghost-like, a very faint memory of themselves, because they are eked out in a medium of all-embracing nonentity. Starches provide an architecture for processed food, just as they help construct paper, glue and industrial lubricants – and we don't expect to eat those. One company sums up the whole purpose of modified starches:

> They are used as bland-tasting functional ingredients in the food industry as fillers, stabilisers, thickeners, pastes, and glues in dry soup mixes, infant foods, sauces, gravy mixes, etc.

You can almost sense the lack of inspiration of the person who wrote that description, struggling to find something positive to say about such a tedious ingredient.

Even the companies that make starches don't attempt to sell their organoleptic qualities. To do so would be a waste of time, because all food manufacturers understand that they taste, at best, of zilch. Instead, they try to make a virtue out of nothingness. 'The bland taste of potato starches allows whole meat products to maintain their natural palatability' is how one starch company puts it. A more forthright version of the same message might read 'the boringness of starch won't interfere with other ingredients', and a postscript might add 'but they will most certainly pad them out.'

And if the addition of starch means a net loss in flavour, it almost always translates into a net loss of nutrition also, because when highly refined starches of the type used in food manufacture replace proteins, fats, and fruits and vegetables, they actually worsen the nutritional profile of the resulting products. More starch in a recipe means less of some other ingredient, and in most cases, that other ingredient was a damn sight more nutritious.

Now this might sound counterintuitive if you have paid attention to the standard government nutrition advice: 'Rather than avoiding starchy foods, it's better to try and base your meals on them, so they make up about a third of your diet.' In recent times, starchy foods, even the most refined types, have been hyped by public health agencies. Starchy foods, such as cereals, pasta and bread, we are told, 'are a good source of energy and the main source of a range of nutrients in our diet. As well as starch, they contain fibre, calcium, iron and B vitamins'. This presentation of starchy carbohydrate as a hero nutrient is highly debatable. If we are going to champion certain foods on the basis of micronutrients, such as iron and B vitamins, then meat would be a better bet because it contains them in greater abundance. As for fibre, we can get all we need from vegetables and fruit.

Of course, starchy carbs in their whole, unprocessed forms do contain some useful micronutrients, but the same cannot be said for the refined sort, which would be more accurately described as stodge, or fodder. Refined starches are rapidly broken down into simple sugars and readily absorbed into the bloodstream. This is why, if you chew a bit of white bread for a few seconds longer than usual, it will begin to taste sweet. Refined carbohydrates cause spikes in our blood sugar and insulin levels, which encourages our bodies to produce and store fat. Long term, this predisposes us to chronic disease. Due to their smaller particle size, highly processed, chemically or physically altered starches – precisely the type used in food processing – cause an even faster rise in blood sugar. So when food manufacturers brag about reducing sugar – on the surface, a noble mission – it is worthwhile noting that if starch is the replacement, then this is a case of more of the same. Think of it as a gesture, a tactical, piecemeal reformulation that should not be mistaken for a radical one.

In so many ways, starch is a never-ending source of inspiration to food manufacturers. Classless starch finds a role in every echelon of food processing, everything from stiffening an up-market reduced fat crème fraiche, to putting a shine on a down-market gravy. Its facelessness allows it to go everywhere and anywhere. Using starch, food manufacturers can even concoct products that defy the fundamental principles of food preparation. The example of mayonnaise comes to mind. In its traditional incarnation, the recipe requires only two ingredients: oil and egg yolk. A touch of salt, vinegar or lemon juice can be added, but they are not essential; oil and egg yolk whisked into a natural emulsion is, in itself, a pleasurable thing to eat. Here, for comparison, are the ingredients of an Asda Extra Light Mayonnaise:

> Water, Spirit Vinegar, Sugar, Modified Maize Starch, Vegetable Oil (5.5%), Pasteurised Salted Free Range Egg Yolk (4.5%) [Pasteurised Free Range Egg Yolk, Salt], Dijon Mustard [Water, Mustard Seeds, Spirit Vinegar, Salt, Preservative (Potassium Metabisulphite), Acidity Regulator (Citric Acid)], Salt, Maltodextrin, Acidity Regulator (Lactic Acid), Colour (Titanium Dioxide), Stabiliser (Guar Gum), Preservative (Potassium Sorbate), Antioxidant (Calcium Disodium Ethylene)]

Instead of two ingredients, you have twenty. Sugar, salt and vinegar cover in taste terms for the paucity of egg and the generous volume of water. A 'light', low-fat tag dangles the promise of improved health, while the choice of feel-good free-range egg strategically draws attention away from feel-bad, rough and redneck spirit vinegar, and a whole gang of additives. This and many other clever concoctions are only made possible by the uniting presence of starch. No wonder food manufacturers are glued to the stuff.

12

Tricky

The use of chemicals in food processing doesn't go down well with the general public. Manufacturers know this, hence the general food industry shift to 'clean label' products that appear to contain only natural, recognisable ingredients you would find in a domestic larder.

The odd bit of information that comes our way about less visible chemical techniques used behind the scenes of food processing – and it is the very odd bit because such information needn't be disclosed on product labels – is often disturbing. Who wants to think that the oil they are cooking with was stripped from seeds using the toxic solvent, hexane, or degummed using caustic soda? Who licks their lips when they learn that the centre of their chocolate cherry stays liquid because the sugar was processed using corrosive hydrochloric acid? And what should we do with such knowledge? Stop eating processed food entirely?

Most of us crave a less radical solution. Can't scientists come up with a more benign way to give us the range of processed foods that we have become accustomed to? A hi-tech magic bullet that would take factory food into a new, improved, more civilised era, sweeping away all the persistent health and environmental concerns that attach to old, unpopular chemical treatments?

If you believe certain not disinterested voices in the food industry, such a solution already exists. Enzymes, we are told, are one of the leading 'green chemistry' technologies, designed to reduce or eliminate generations of hazardous substances that have now fallen from grace. According to the European Food Information Council, a body 'supported by companies of the European food and drinks industries' to convey science-based information to the public' – in other words, an industry lobby group – 'enzymes make clean, green food'.

If your grasp of chemistry is shaky, the word enzyme might cause you to stumble. In simple terms, enzymes are proteins that occur naturally in the cells of plants, animals and microorganisms. They are essential to the metabolism of all living things. The human body, for example, uses enzymes to carry out many biochemical processes, such as digestion. The names of most, but not all, enzymes end in 'ase', as in amylase, protease.

In commercial terms, enzymes are best known for their industrial applications. They are used, for example, to make laundry and dishwashing detergents, for stone-washing jeans, in pulp and paper manufacture, for leather de-hairing and tanning, in de-sizing of textiles and de-inking paper, to make contact lens cleaner, and for the degreasing of cattle hides. But don't let any of that put you off enzymes in your food and drink. Here, the Enzyme Technical Association, a trade association of companies that make and market enzyme products, explains the 'enzyme advantage':

> The use of enzymes frequently results in many benefits that cannot be obtained with traditional chemical treatment. These often include higher product quality and lower manufacturing cost, less waste and reduced energy consumption. More traditional chemical treatments are generally nonspecific, not always easily controlled, and may create harsh conditions. Often they produce undesirable side effects and/or waste disposal problems.

What's not to like? Food manufacturers are certainly convinced that enzymes are the way forward. They have embraced enzyme technology to such an extent that nowadays, nearly all commercially prepared foods contain at least one ingredient that has been made with them. Enzymes are already widely used in the production of sugar syrups, starches, artificial sweeteners, bakery products, soft and alcoholic drinks, instant breakfast cereals, cereal-based baby foods, cheese, dairy and egg products (such as dried egg powder), fruit juice, instant noodles, vegetable oil, confectionery, meat tenderising brines, flavourings and instant coffee. New trademarked enzyme products are coming onto the market all the time.

Food manufacturers use enzymes as catalysts, triggers to speed up chemical reactions that would otherwise proceed very slowly, or in some cases, not happen at all. There are millions of enzymes in nature, and they act quickly: some of them perform their task up to five million times a minute. So enzymes work all sorts of magic and make many products feasible that would otherwise never pass Go. Enzymes, in the words of companies active in the field, do 'the work of a small factory'.

By using certain amylases during fermentation, for instance, brewers can make low calorie beers. Most of the controversial sweetener, high fructose corn syrup (HFCS), which finds its way into soft drinks, sweets, baking, jams and jellies and many other foods, is now produced using enzymes, such as alpha-amylase. To ensure that bakery goods, such as breakfast bars, and sweets maintain desirably soft, chewy centres for weeks at a time when otherwise they would harden, manufacturers use invertase. Amyloglucosidase will give industrial bread an evenly brown crust, while maltogenic amylase will delay the rate at which it stales. Industrial baking plants often use a mix of enzymes – typically three to five at a time – in most or all of their products, on a daily basis. A dash of pectin methylesterase will make your frozen raspberries and green beans firmer.

Many of the flavours we come across in familiar cheeses – Cheddar, mozzarella, Parmesan, Emmental, cream cheese – are not due to the intrinsic taste of local milk, or to patient maturation and flavour development, but to the action of man-made enzymes called lipases that are added during the ripening stage of production. In order to make a juice that is crystal clear rather than cloudy, manufacturers will process the juice with pectinase. This enzyme is also used to treat citrus fruits before they are made into marmalade, or candied, and to extract the very last little bit of juice from grapes by breaking down their cell walls before they are made into wine. Pectinase firms up fruits and vegetables so that they retain their shape better during processing. If, for instance, you have ever eaten one of those yogurts that has a layer of fruit at the bottom with whole, more intact strawberries rather than just a purée, those berries could have been treated with pectinase.

To strengthen them before the processing onslaught, the strawberries, fresh or frozen, could have been incubated in a solution of calcium chloride, a salt more commonly used for ice and dust control on roads, to which the enzyme has been added. One company that makes such an enzyme product says that it increases the firmness of the fruit or vegetable, improves what manufacturers call 'fruit integrity' during processing, and extends the shelf life of soft fruit. Fresh peeled citrus fruit segments destined for ready-to-eat fruit salads are often processed with pectinase to give them a better texture and appearance.

If some of these uses of enzymes sound like more of a boon to the manufacturers than the consumer, rest assured that the same can be said for many enzyme products. For instance, one type of maltogenic amylase for bakery is marketed as VERON® xTender – 'The Extra Tender Shelf-life Extender', which sums up all you really need to know about its purpose. A protease enzyme, Maxipro HSP, won the coveted prize for the Savoury/Meat Innovation of the Year Award at the Food Ingredients Europe Excellence Awards, for its ability to extract protein from animal by-products, such as blood. DSM, the company that makes it, explains:

> With Maxipro HSP, our radically new enzyme solution, the industry is able to capture the nutritional and commercial value of blood side streams by recovering all the available protein, enabling a more sustainable production of processed meat products. MaxiPro HSP has proven to be particularly efficient in removing the heme part from the blood protein hemoglobin. This heme group is responsible for the red-to-dark brown color and the iron taste, making

> hemoglobin difficult to apply in high end meat applications ... The result is a more effective decolorisation process that preserves the valuable functionalities of the globin protein, while selectively removing the strong taste and dark odor of the heme.

You can see why this enzyme product is feted by manufacturers of low-grade meat products. The global meat industry is ever keen to maximise the potential of its by-products, and DSM says that Maxipro HSP has 'excellent gelation and waterbinding properties'. But it's a rare consumer who really relishes the thought of enzyme-treated blood in their bangers.

Subtilisin is another enzyme employed to reinvent red blood cells as a usable ingredient. It produces a purified product that 'may be spray-dried and is used in cured meats, sausages and luncheon meats'.

Enzymes reach right down the food chain to the farm and the slaughterhouse. Many animal feedstuffs are treated with phytases, carbohydrases and proteases. One feed enzymes company commentator explains their purpose:

> Animal feed is the largest cost item in livestock and poultry production, accounting for 60–70 per cent of total expenses. To save on costs, many producers supplement feed with enzyme additives, which enable them to produce more meat per animal or to produce the same amount of meat cheaper and faster.

The phrase 'cheaper and faster' is always music to the ears of producers of intensively reared meat.

Enzymes cut farmers' costs because they can use less protein in the feed, and protein is expensive to buy. One enzyme company boasts that chickens fed a two per cent lower protein diet supplemented with a protease enzyme grew as large as birds that were fed a standard diet containing more protein. Enzymes also improve the profile of cheaper animal feeds, such as feather meal. A by-product of processing poultry, it is made by processing feathers, using heat and pressure, grinding them, and drying them. This type of feed is used in fish farming as a cheap, low-rent alternative to fish meal. But it does have an image problem, as BioResource International, a feed enzyme company explains:

> It is widely known that feather meal – as an alternative to expensive fish meal – is one way for animal producers to diversify their feed protein sources. However, feather meal use is limited by the perception that it is poorly digested, not as balanced, and is of poor quality. True. True. And true. But that was then. Today, BRI's Valkerase® can take your underperforming, poorly digested feather meal and turn it into a more optimised source of digestible proteins and peptides that rivals that of other protein sources.

Mmmm, anyone fancy a fillet of farmed salmon or rainbow trout?

At the abattoir, proteases do the job of recovering protein from the skeletons of animals and fish after butchering or filleting, as one company explains: 'Material recovered using proteases can be produced from coarse and fine scrap-bone residues from the mechanical fleshing of beef, pig, turkey, or chicken bones.' Using such enzymes, a further five per cent of the adhering flesh can be removed – sucked, scraped or otherwise mechanically extracted – from the bones or cartilage. The process for extracting every last little bit of protein isn't one for faint hearts. The carcasses are mashed and incubated in hot water with the enzymes for several hours. 'The meat slurry produced', one authority explains, 'is used in canned meats and soups'. Waste not, want not.

There are other more direct ways to use enzymes for meat. Older, lower value animals, such as unproductive dairy cows, whose less than prime flesh would otherwise be tough, can be injected with a type of papain enzyme directly into the jugular vein shortly before slaughter; this has the effect of tenderising their meat.

Over 150 enzymes are now used by the food and drink industry. News to you? And to most people. As the Enzyme Technical Association reflects, 'the importance of enzymes in everyday life is one of today's best-kept secrets'. But why don't we know more about their extensive use? After all, some enzymes, notably those used in starch processing and high-fructose syrup manufacture, are now traded as commodity products on the world's markets, so global financial markets are fully aware of them, even if most citizens are in the dark about their very existence.

The simple answer to this question is that because enzymes are so powerful and effective in their action, the amount needed to accomplish the desired effect is small, usually 0.1 per cent, or less, of a product's overall composition. It is assumed that enzymes used in food and drink manufacture are generally deactivated or used up during processing, and therefore not present in the final food product. Enzyme companies successfully lobbied for a regulatory distinction between what food is produced *from* and what it is produced *with*, and regulators agreed to treat enzymes as processing aids: 'they shall be present in the food in the form of a residue, if at all, and shall have no technological effect on the finished product'. Under European law, processing aids don't need to be labelled. Fresh efforts by the European Commission to revisit the classification of enzymes are under way, but as one industry consultant points out: 'The industry will kick and scream if that vast majority of enzymes are not in fact regulated as processing aids.' For the time being, unless enzymes are used as additives – and hardly any are – you won't see them on the product label.

It might strike you that there could conceivably be an important qualitative difference between enzymes that occur naturally, such as those found in human saliva, or in our guts, and those that are made commercially in a factory. These man-made enzyme preparations are used out of their original contexts to drive chemical reactions. Indeed, the processes used to extract and isolate enzymes for commercial use increases their effect. The European Food Information Council explains the potency of these factory-made enzyme products: 'Purified enzymes do not lose their properties, on the contrary, these 'cell-free' preparations work even more efficiently.'

The enzymes used in food processing are obtained in very particular ways. Many of them are now developed using genetic modification (GM) techniques. Genetic engineering is bringing new enzymes to market all the time, as the European Commission explains:

> Due to new technologies, new enzymes not accessible before can be cloned into and produced from a well-known host organism. Thereby, enzymes from almost any source in nature become accessible, including enzymes exhibiting unusual properties, such as extreme thermostability [stability in heat].

Ultimately, the European Commission points out, new technologies such as GM 'might lead to enzymes not present in nature so far'. Depending on your philosophical approach to food technology, this might, or might not, sound like the plot line of a sci-fi horror story. Already, some of the most common enzymes in our food are GM. Their uses include catalase (for mayonnaise), chymosin (for cheese-making), beta-glucanase (in brewing), xylanase (in baking) and lipase (in oils). More and more commercial enzymes are made by GM methods these days, because genetic engineering makes it easier to produce them on an industrial scale.

Yet there is widespread ignorance that GM enzymes are used at all. If a manufacturer were to include a GM ingredient in a food or drink, under European law it would have to be labelled as such. The reason only a handful of foods in the UK contain GM ingredients is because when people see GM on the ingredients listing, they don't want to buy the product. But because GM enzymes don't need to be declared, citizens are not given a similar opportunity to reject them.

GM or otherwise, the enzymes used to make food and drink are manufactured from microorganisms, animal organs, and material such as fungi. For instance lipase, an enzyme used to make cheese, bread, dried egg white and protein powders, can be made from animal pancreatic tissue, certain types of Aspergillus mould, or the stomach tissue of calves, kids or lambs. Asparaginase, used in the manufacture of potato chips, crisps, biscuits, crackers and breakfast cereal, is made from *Escherichia coli*, a bacterium better known for being found in the lower intestine of warm-blooded organisms. As Andrew Whitley, Britain's foremost authority on artisan baking, puts it:

> For the food enzyme industry, all of nature is a chemistry set. No organisms are too exotic or repulsive to be investigated for possible active agents.

The catholic collection of substances from which commercial enzymes may be harvested should clearly raise ethical issues. Observant Muslims, Jews and vegans would be horrified to learn, for instance, that the phospholipase used to make their bread was once derived from pig's pancreas. They need never know, however, because neither the presence of enzymes, nor their source material, need be disclosed.

Once the raw materials are sourced, how are commercial enzymes made? The production involves large-scale fermentation in tanks with capacities of up to 150,000 litres. The contents are referred to in the enzyme business as a 'broth'. But what is in the recipe? The European Commission observes: 'Details of components used in industrial-scale fermentation broths for enzyme production are not readily obtained. Not surprisingly, as manufacturers do not wish to reveal information that may be of technical or commercial value to their competitors.' As for ordinary people, if the regulators are struggling, we haven't a hope in hell of discovering what went into the enzyme soup. Likely ingredients, however, are waste materials and by-products from the food and agricultural industries, materials as diverse as sugars, sulphite liquid from cellulose production plants, hydrolysed [chemically broken down] wood and starch, fruit juices, potatoes, phosphates, soya meal, dairy, meat and vegetable proteins, derivatives of ammonia, cotton seed, corn-steeping liquid and fish meal. Usually, the raw materials are dissolved or suspended in water, and heated. The enzymes are secreted into the fermented broth.

From the broth stage, the disrupted cells go through further purification steps. The European Commission describes these as follows in its usual all-embracing, comprehensive manner: 'A variety of chemical, mechanical and thermal [heat] techniques (concentration, precipitation, extraction, centrifugation, filtration, chromatography).' The resulting enzyme concentrate is then sold to food and drink companies in various forms – liquids, slurries, granules and powders – depending on what is required, preparations that contain additives to stabilise the enzyme activity and act as preservatives.

Need the soupy, hazy pedigree of the enzymes used to make our food and drink cause us any concern? The enzyme industry would argue that we should continue to enjoy the fruits of enzyme technology without a care in the world. But how much confidence should that give us? Bear in mind the cautionary tale of azodicarbonamide and potassium bromate. For decades, bakers were shovelling these chemical additives into their products, on the basis that they had been granted Generally Regarded As Safe (GRAS) status from regulators. Belatedly, European regulators got round to banning them when the scientific case against them became too glaring to ignore. The former was linked to respiratory problems, allergies and asthma; the latter is thought to be carcinogenic. Both of these have been replaced by – guess what? – supposedly safer enzymes. Safe for how long? As artisan baking expert Andrew Whitley wryly observes, 'safety assurance has a short shelf life'.

Can we trust that factory-made enzymes are safe? The enzyme industry's tight-lipped lack of transparency doesn't exactly build confidence. When the European Commission asked the Austrian Federal Environment Agency to assemble a collection of information on enzymes, the research team made a point of noting tactfully in its final report the lack of co-operation it had received from enzyme companies:

> The project team explicitly acknowledges the efforts made by some individual representatives of industry to provide information, however, also regrets not having received all data requested from industry.

The team notes how initially, 'co-operation with industry was very promising' but ultimately, even after giving the industry more time to supply data that would answer its questions, 'these data were not provided by industry'. So the project team had to base its conclusions mainly on relatively limited data available from other sources. On key issues, such as whether genetic engineering has different impacts on the properties of enzymes, the team pointed out that available data sources were 'very narrow'.

It is well known that enzymes can trigger health problems in people. Biological 'bio' washing powders, for example, can cause skin irritation. Itchy skin is relatively trivial, but as potential allergens, enzymes can have more dramatic effects if inhaled as a dust. Enzymes are a well-documented occupational hazard for those who work in industrial bakeries; workers in such environments are usually screened for allergies and respiratory problems, and having passed these checks, are required to wear protective clothing and impervious gauntlet gloves. Once an individual has developed an immune response to the enzyme, re-exposure produces increasingly severe responses that can be dangerous or even fatal. What begins as a runny nose, or soreness of the fingertips, can develop into breathing difficulties and, in rare cases, severe anaphylactic shock, which can prove fatal. This is why dry, dusty enzyme preparations are being replaced by liquid or granular ones where the enzymes are said to be 'immobilised'. Even so, enzyme companies usually recommend to food and drink manufacturers that employees working with liquid enzymes use eye protection to avoid splashes.

What effects might enzymes have on people who eat and drink products made with them? Potential impacts on the health of consumers of such products, as well as the people who make them, cannot be ruled out. European Commission researchers point out that although there is at present no evidence of reactions to eating enzymes in food, in theory, such sensitisation could occur. What's more, many enzymes have been specifically designed to remain highly stable during the heat and stress of food and drink production processes, which means that they 'could more easily pass through the intestine without being fully degraded or denatured'. One such example is fungal alpha-amylase: a study has found that 20 per cent of its allergenicity can survive in the crusts of bread. Another example is transglutaminase, which is used in bread and pastries, such as croissants, to make the dough more elastic, and also to bond low-quality meat products. One group of researchers has found that it can generate the epitope [part of molecule] responsible for coeliac disease. Proteases, a class of enzymes that makes particularly effective detergent, are commonly used in industrial baking and for meat tenderising. These are the most likely to cause allergies and sensitivities because they have the easiest access to the bloodstream through soft tissues.

It is also theoretically possible that allergenic enzymes, even if not present in the final product, could contaminate the factories where they are used. The vast majority of product recalls that food manufacturers are forced to make concern conventional allergens, such as nuts and soya, which have lingered on in the wrong place at the wrong time. Even with the most scrupulous manufacturing precautions, allergens have a habit of turning up like the proverbial bad penny, because they are difficult to control in an industrial plant environment.

Allergies apart, no enzyme has yet been shown to be toxic, mutagenic or carcinogenic, but it is accepted that residual contaminants, derived from the enzyme source itself, or produced during processing, such as mycotoxins and aflatoxins, could be a health hazard. In the USA, enzymes must have Generally Regarded As Safe (GRAS) status, for what that's worth. In the UK, enzymes used in food are classed as 'substances that the available evidence suggests are acceptable for use in food'. Note that mealy-mouthed, damage-limiting, covering-my-back phrase 'available evidence suggests'. As we know from the experience of the team tasked by the European Commission with collecting data on enzymes, not enough information is available to draw deeply informed conclusions. It is almost as if regulators have been unable to keep up with the speed at which enzymes are being developed, or form a full picture of their long-term implications.

For legislative purposes, commercial enzymes are treated as 'natural'. Any testing that has taken place is narrow and restrictive, looking at each enzyme in isolation with an obstinate tunnel vision. No serious attention has been given to the fact that enzymes, most notably in baking, are often used in compound mixes of up to five at a time, along with other chemical additives, and coyly named as 'improvers'. What might the cocktail effect of such enzyme and chemical mixes be? How might they multiply the allergen and toxin risk? No regulatory body appears to have given this any serious consideration.

But why should this cause us a minute's concern? Speaking for enzyme companies, the European Food Information Council argues that 'the concept of acceptable risk is intrinsic to the notion of pushing back the frontiers [of science]'. Of course, the issue for most people is, 'Do I and my family really want to be part of a human experiment at the cutting edge of enzyme technology?' Don't spend too long thinking about that question. You aren't being consulted on the question, and so, to all intents and purposes, your opinion doesn't matter.

13

Old

The word 'fresh' can be relied upon to conjure up positive images. Used honestly and accurately, it is an epithet that fits the perky greenness of recently harvested vegetables, a handful of cut herbs from the garden, or fruit just picked in the orchard. It conveys the sense of food prepared and consumed the same day, without any refrigeration: newly fired pizza, a Sunday dinner cooked in the late afternoon and eaten in the early evening, a just-baked scone, a stir-fry hot from the wok. At a stretch, fresh can describe ingredients that have been lightly processed: a kipper still warm from the smokehouse, even a pat of newly churned butter. Yet the word 'fresh' is used by food retailers and manufacturers in an entirely different way: to refer to products that have undergone some treatment to prolong their edible life.

If you stop to think about it, this usage is a contradiction in terms. 'Fresh' is, or ought to be, time sensitive. By its very nature, freshness is a fleeting and finite state, a concept located at the top end of a timescale that inevitably leads downwards to decomposition and decay. For food manufacturers and retailers, however, the word 'fresh' has assumed an obligingly elastic meaning. They sell us chilled food and drink under the banner of fresh – ready meals, dips, salads, sandwiches, fried fish, soups, smoothies, cooked meats, spreads, cook-in sauces, pizza, desserts, chicken nuggets – and give it a use-by date that leads us to believe that they will stay like this for days at a time.

By rights, the confused notion of fresh food that lasts some considerable time should be oxymoronic, but in food manufacture, freshness has become synonymous with a more truthful, accurate term: 'shelf-life extension'. A number of more and less sophisticated technologies have been developed with the sole purpose of making food last longer. As a consequence old, tired food masquerading as fresh has become a big part of our diet.

Over 80 additives that have a preservative effect are approved in Europe. Each has an E number, the tell-tale badge that indicates to consumers they are man-made. The chemical industry tries doggedly to convince us that any instinctive hostility to such preservatives merely reflects the scientific illiteracy of the general public. The Food Additives and Ingredients Association (FAIA, http://www.faia.org.uk), a body representing chemical companies that make these additives, attempts to relax us by telling us that many of them are just 'synthetic copies of the natural [preservative] products that are present in nature'. If we only understood more about them, we wouldn't be so reluctant to consume them, we're told. So what are they?

First up are those classed as preservatives: benzoates (such as sodium benzoate, sodium ethyl p-hydroxybenzoate), nitrites and nitrates (such as potassium nitrite, sodium nitrate), sorbates (such as sodium sorbate, potassium sorbate), sulfites (such as potassium metabisulfite), and propionates (such as calcium propionate, propionic acid). This class of preservative turns up in many products, from muffins, through processed meats and mango juice, to milkshakes.

Clearly, this motley crew doesn't go down too well with the 'no chemicals brigade' – a food industry term of derision for people who routinely avoid additives and obscure ingredients with unfamiliar names. Such preservatives are, as one food engineer tactfully puts it, 'quite chemical in nature', and the fact that they can cause health problems is beyond dispute. The additive industry itself admits that sulfites, and benzoic acid and its derivatives, can trigger breathing difficulties, shortness of breath, wheezing and coughing in sensitive individuals. Strong evidence suggests that consumption of the preservative sodium benzoate, in tandem with certain artificial food colours, could be linked to increased hyperactivity in children. These relatively minor reactions pale into insignificance when you consider the well-recorded impacts of the nitrates that have become standard kit in processed meats. Converted by bacteria in saliva to nitrates, these then react with various amines in the stomach to form nitrosamines, which are potent carcinogens.

Next in line in the assembled ranks of shelf-life extenders are antioxidants. These might appear more benign than the preservatives mentioned above, even beneficial, because relatively few people appreciate that they are quite a different kettle of fish from the natural antioxidants in raw food that disarm cell damage-causing free radicals. Ascorbic acid is the personable ambassador thrust forward to speak for this category, and regularly introduced as vitamin C by another name. But this is misleading. Ascorbic acid is made industrially in factories, often by the fermentation of GM corn, by triggering a series of chemical reactions. So the ascorbic acid that draws attention away from the woeful nutritional profile of fruit 'drinks', or nutrient-denuded breakfast cereals and breads, is a one-dimensional, man-made copy of natural vitamin C found in whole foods, such as oranges and kale. While vitamin C in real food is always accompanied by other micronutrients that act in synergy to enhance its effect, ascorbic acid is an isolated, man-made chemical, and as such, is unlikely to have the same health-boosting effects as natural vitamin C. The same reservation applies to another group of antioxidants, tocopherols: alpha-tocopherol, gamma-tocopherol, delta-tocopherol, mixed tocopherols. These chemically manipulated, synthesised versions of natural vitamin E are usually derived from petrol. Synthetic vitamins are not as well absorbed in the body as natural ones.

The antioxidant line-up looks uglier still when you glimpse other lower profile personalities skulking in the ranks, additives that turn up like clockwork in crisps, crackers, chips, margarine, processed meats, and foods fried in oil, such as chicken Kievs, falafels and fish fingers. Meet butylated hydroxytoluene (BHT), which is also an ingredient in embalming fluid and jet fuel, butylated hydroxyanisole (BHA), a common component of rubber and petroleum products, propyl gallate, often used to make glues, and tert-butylhydroquinone (TBHQ), which finds another purpose in the making of varnish. A lively scientific debate surrounds these antioxidants because several studies have found they have adverse effects on laboratory animals – cancer, disruption to hormones and the nervous system, and more. However, in their infinite wisdom, our regulators have concluded that the presence of these additives, at the levels permitted, represents no risk to human health. The need of food processors to postpone the evil hour when their products start showing their age trumps public health concerns every time.

You can see why acronyms are necessary – these additive names don't exactly trip off the tongue. Nor do they inspire consumer confidence. And why should they? The knowledge that many food additives have the capacity to shorten the lives of humans, as well as extend use-by dates, is built into European law. This is why regulators have set a maximum 'acceptable daily intake' for each one, based on the 'no-observed-adverse-effect level' which, we are told, is a 'safe' limit based on animal experiments. Researchers observe what dose laboratory animals can take of a substance before showing obvious signs of illness, or dying, and then extrapolate from this the likely effects on humans. But this is an informed estimate; no one really knows how much of a carcinogen it takes to cause cancer, or how much of a toxin it takes to poison your nervous system.

According to the European Food Information Council (EUFIC) – a body that presents itself as a 'science-based' information body on food, but which functions as a food industry lobby group – acceptable daily intakes include 'a large margin of safety and refers to the amount of a food additive that can be taken daily in the diet, over a lifetime span, without any negative effect on health'. Fine and dandy, if you take on trust assurances from the food industry's men in white coats, but then many of us don't. The public appetite for an alphabet soup of additives has shrunk.

Much more effective in softening up doubting consumers has been the fiction, fostered by the processed food industry, that the main reason for using preservative additives is to make foods safer. In this storyline, preservatives are presented as front-line fighters protecting us from poisoning and death. This is how the EUFIC frames the argument:

> The greatest threat to consumers is that of food being spoiled, or from becoming toxic by the effect of micro-organisms (e.g. bacteria, yeast, moulds) occurring in them. Some of these organisms can secrete poisonous substances ('toxins'), which are dangerous to human health and can even be fatal.

This 'use a toxin to kill a toxin' propaganda has been tacitly reinforced by the health and safety establishment. It has groomed us to see natural, unprocessed food as a seething mass of sinister bacteria that can only be rendered safe by the controlling hand of technology. Case in point, under the tabloid-style headline 'Kitchen sink squalor', NHS Choices warns us that 'most people think of the toilet as the most contaminated part of the house, but in fact the kitchen sink typically contains 100,000 times more germs than a bathroom or lavatory'. Scary or what? This is typical of the tone of government food hygiene advice, wherein home cooks are portrayed as dangerously ignorant, exposing their nearest and dearest to life-threatening hazards. In government food hygiene campaigns, no mention is made of the much more extensive food poisoning risks routinely run in factory food production, or of how the modern food distribution system can facilitate the spread of a problem to thousands of homes, thousands of miles away, in a matter of hours.

The effect of this slanted emphasis on domestic food poisoning risk is to undermine the confidence of home cooks in our ability to prepare safe food. It makes us crave the apparent safety of processed, manufactured food and drink. In the opinion of one Twitter correspondent, 'A factory is what we call a hygienic, efficient place to prepare food. It's safer than a farmhouse kitchen.' Such sentiment is widespread amongst generations that have never learned to cook and so are heavily dependent on processed food and takeaways. Bring on those protective additives please! But the truth of the matter is that with the exception of the nitrate and nitrite preservatives used in cured meats such as bacon, there is no overarching food safety reason to use preservatives or antioxidants in fresh food, unless, that is, you want to extend its natural life. And that, quite candidly, is the main function of preservative additives in processed food: to feed the illusion that food is fresher, and newer, than it actually is. Why bother? There's money in it, as one purveyor of 'shelf-life enhancement solutions' says: 'The ability to extend the shelf life of a food or beverage is all-important for manufacturers and retailers. By extending shelf life, the profitability is directly impacted in a positive direction.' If that sounds a bit woolly, this balder reasoning from another such company makes the financial motivation a whole lot clearer: 'There are no improvements that you can make to your food or beverage product that will boost your customer [retailer] satisfaction and increase your bottom line as much as shelf-life extension.'

Supermarkets constantly lean on manufacturers to put longer 'best before' dates on chilled products. This helps to feed the consumer myth they encourage that it isn't necessary to shop fairly frequently for food if you want it to be fresh. In 2013, Kathryn Callaghan, from the UK FSA's Hygiene and Microbiology Division, warned the Royal Society for Public

Health that 'in the past 20 years, there has been an increasing trend' for longer shelf life. She was talking in the context of ready-to-eat meats, one of the highest food poisoning risk categories, and said: 'I actually visited a couple of smaller manufacturers and they told us there's a lot of pressure on them ... to put a long shelf life on their products.'

Appreciating that it is losing the argument with consumers over E number additives, and keen to be seen to be responding to 'clean label' pressure from supermarkets, and driven by the desire for a long shelf life, the processed food industry has come up with newer techniques to make 'fresh' food last longer in less obvious ways. The name of the game is to lose artificial additives and replace them with those that sound more natural, but to do so is technically challenging. In the absence of straight like-for-like substitutes, manufacturers are adopting a belt and braces approach, using modern cocktails of shelf life-stretching substances to produce the desired effect, often in tandem with modified atmosphere packaging (MAP).

Few of us notice the now extensive use of this preservation method in the chilled food aisles. By altering the composition of air in plastic packs so that it contains significantly less, or no, oxygen, MAP keeps all sorts of 'fresh' products looking young longer, just like Sleeping Beauty, who went to sleep for years but woke up exactly the same age. In conjunction with refrigeration, MAP is the technological fix that allows the surface of meat to remain ruby red when otherwise it would darken. It prevents young cheeses from developing moulds and stops ready-to-cook vegetables from appearing dry. In packs flushed with MAP, sliced meats and 'fresh' pasta won't curl up at the edges. The breath of air you feel as you peel open a wedge of Parmesan, a bag of grated cheese, or a lunchtime salad bowl? That's modified atmosphere.

MAP used to be a technology that was utterly invisible. Now foods packaged using MAP must be labelled. In the tiniest writing, eagle-eyed consumers will spot the cosseting phrase 'packaged in a protective atmosphere'. This form of words is a classic case of the processed food industry presenting its intervention in a favourable light. Alternative terminologies for MAP in the trade are 'gas-flushed', 'gas-packaged', 'gas-shocked', or even plain old 'gassed', but they don't sound so nurturing.

Compared to preservative chemicals, MAP is low down the list of consumer concerns. Many of us find it handy to have one of those stiff packets of pitta breads as a stand-by; few appreciate that they are packed in modified air. Using MAP, pre-baked pitta breads, and for that matter, bagels, wraps and tortillas stored at room temperature will see an increase in shelf life from around 5 to 20 days. Some bakery goods can be given a shelf life of up to 6 months if so packaged. MAP can add 5 or 6 days to the shelf life of a sandwich; just the job for petrol station forecourts and corner shops with a sluggish trade.

Sealed in a modified atmosphere, the use-by date of a ready meal can be increased from between 2 and 5 days to between 5 and 10 days. Few of us would put a home-cooked meal in the fridge and eat it 10 days later; we would worry that it was too old. But a factory-made ready meal flushed with MAP can reach that age and still seem fresh. And bear in mind that the meat and fish in many processed foods – things like chicken salads, prawn sandwiches, chicken tikka, battered fish fillets – will more than likely have been bought by the manufacturer frozen, defrosted for the production process, and then sent out, gas-flushed and chilled, as 'fresh'. Working out the age of many of the component ingredients in processed food would require the services of a very sharp detective, if not Interpol, but it is fair to assume that key ingredients are a whole lot less youthful than we like to think.

MAP performs another service to ready meal manufacturers: it delays the onset of what is known in the factory food trade as 'warmed over flavour' or WOF, an off-taste likened to 'damp dog hair' that develops in pre-cooked fish, meat and poultry. Think of the heated caskets or 'coffins' filled with tepid meals that are sent out to hospitals and schools from far distant institutional kitchens, overlay it with the wet cardboard odour that hangs around a box of breaded fish that has spent too long in the freezer, add a pinch of trace metals from factory cooking and processing equipment, and you have a whiff of it.

At the typical supermarket 'butcher's' counter, no real butchery takes place. What's on sale will most likely have arrived from the abattoir cutting line as pre-cut, 'case ready' meat in large containers filled with modified air. Meat imported frozen to the UK from abroad, New Zealand lamb for instance, can be defrosted at a processing plant, then flushed with MAP. Why? Counter staff don't need to be properly trained butchers and it buys the retailer time, as one company active in MAP technology explains: 'Using the correct modified atmosphere packaging conditions, shelf life of red meat can typically be increased from around 2–4 days to between 5 and 8 days under refrigeration, while that of poultry can be increased from 4–7 days to 16–21 days'.

Chopped up chicken that's 3 weeks old? It's not the acme of freshness or food safety, but then no one in the food processing business dreams for one minute that it is, as Dansensor, a company specialising in MAP, makes plain:

> The driving force behind this distinctive gas packaging trend is the combination of a strong consumer appeal (fresh products) and a number of benefits to the retailers in connection with logistics, product presentation, value added products, extended food shelf life etc. The purpose of gas flushed packaging is to give the product a long shelf life.

More often than not, MAP is used to disguise signs of what the food industry calls 'light processing': cleaning, washing, paring, coring and dicing. Whether you're talking pineapple chunks, or microwave-ready broccoli florets, these interventions behind the scenes inevitably make fruits and vegetables more perishable because they disrupt cell tissues and break down cell membranes. In fact, these 'fresh-cut products' as they are known in the business, are what scientists refer to as 'wounded' tissues, so they deteriorate more rapidly than intact fruits and vegetables. MAP is used to delay the obvious signs of trauma – browning and off-flavours – but not always that effectively. Nutritional value is also reduced, but that loss is invisible to the eye.

Of course shelf life is not to be confused with freshness, as many of us discover when we open a puffy, modified atmosphere 'pillow pack' of salad leaves, only to watch them wilt soon after. Using MAP, prepared vegetable suppliers can add up to 8 days to the use-by date of salad leaves. Allowing for the fact that some time will have elapsed between the leaves being picked and then despatched to the processors for cleaning and packing – let's add on another 1–2 days here – it's no surprise that our bagged salads swoon like a Victorian heroine when exposed to natural air. Poor things, they might be as much as 10 days old, and consequently, their vitality and nutrient profile will be more weakened and degraded than we might like to think.

Then again, collapsed salad leaves could be the worse for wear for other reasons. As a prelude to packing, they will have been put through a vigorous washing machine, or a Jacuzzi-style wash tank, designed to ensure lots of agitation. The best scenario here is that they are washed in spring water, a selling point on a minority of products sold by up-market retailers. Most, however, are sloshed around in tap water dosed with chlorine. Fruit acids – citric, tartaric, and more – in either powder or liquid form, are often also included in the mix. The chlorine passes for 'cleaning' and the acids act as a preservative by inhibiting the growth of bacteria. Some companies that consider themselves progressive and go-ahead are dumping the chlorine for fruit acid washes. Not only do they allow a 'no chlorine' claim to impress consumers, they also have another practical advantage, as the maker of one such product explains:

> NatureSeal FS is not adversely affected by the build-up of organic matter (soil, leaves, and other plant matter). This means that there is no need for frequent changes of wash tank water; some processors operate their wash tanks for at least 8 hours before discharging to drain. Chlorine, which is affected by organic matter, requires more frequent re-dosing and hence the danger of imparting taste taints. This requires wash tanks to be discharged and the water to be changed more often.

In other words, in the cloudy world of fruit and vegetable preparation, it's a choice between fresher water dosed frequently with chlorine, or less frequently changed water blended with acids. Either way, it's a far cry from fruit and vegetables washed in the kitchen sink in tap water. But then, we've been trained by the public health establishment to view our own kitchen sinks with suspicion and to see the tired old gassed, chemical-dipped, bought fruits and vegetables as a safer bet.

With their 'before and after' images, the brochures of companies that promote products to extend shelf life to processors are reminiscent of those adverts that illustrate life-changing claims for the transforming effects of hair transplants, or the wrinkle-diminishing capacity of face cream. Grow Green Industries introduces eatFresh-FC, somewhat enigmatically, as an 'antimicrobial mix of synergistic blend of organic components, citrates and antioxidants [sic]', which, it says, 'preserves colour, texture and freshness, and is proven to extend the shelf life of cut and whole fruits, such as strawberries, apples, pears, mango, avocado and various vegetables'. It goes on to illustrate the point visually. It shows two strawberries after 7 days; the one on the left, the control, has not been dipped in eatFresh-FC; the one on the right has. The control looks rotten, the dipped berry looks immaculately luscious. There are kindred images of cut bananas, apples, pears and avocados, with the undipped fruits inevitably looking brown and old compared to their picture-perfect, dipped equivalents. Grow Green Industries recommends this miraculous, age-defying preparation for use in food service – that's ready prepared food for bars, restaurants, takeaways, schools, hospitals and food retailers. Those oddly tasteless cut apple slices that turn up in airline meals and in sandwich bar 'fresh' fruit salads almost certainly owe their considerable keeping properties to such dips.

'Edible coating technologies' don't stop there. Whole 'fresh' fruits and vegetables can be dipped, drenched or sprayed in products such as Semperfresh, described by its makers as a 'combination of sugar esters and other edible ingredients: vegetable oils and plant cellulose'. It coats each fruit in a very thin, invisible, odourless and tasteless film, which 'slows down the ripening process – effectively putting the produce "to sleep".' Semperfresh is recommended for use both pre- and post-harvest, and can help fruit stay fresh 'for up to twice as long'. It is coatings such as this that make our cherries, apples and pears gleam, and give our peppers, cucumbers and aubergines their lustre.

Moving on from coatings, a number of edible films, known in the food preservation business as 'smart' or 'intelligent' films, are now used by food processors and manufacturers in products as diverse as cheesecake, deli meats and pizza. Imperceptible to consumers, they are made up of gummy, sticky substances that inhibit the growth of bacteria, such as starch, cellulose derivatives, chitosan (an indigestible sugar obtained from the carapace of shellfish), alginates (gel-like seaweed substances), fruit puree, milk and soy proteins, egg white and wheat gluten. According to one advocate of this technology, when used on cut fruits, edible films 'can provide a food with a safe product lifetime of as long as two weeks'. A new edible and cook-able meat coating that promises to extend the shelf life for fresh meat by up to 3 days is being tested. The coating is made from 'a reliable source of naturally occurring peptide compounds', and will be transparent, inodorous and unflavoured. One litre of this MeatCoat solution costs €1.53 and is sufficient to coat 13 square metres of meat.

Edible films are frequently used as carriers for a wide range of artificial additives, such as flavourings and colourings, as well as synthetic preservatives, such as benzoic acid, sorbic acid, propionic acid, lactic acid and nisin. Their presence also slows down the build-up of warmed-over flavour (WOF). Wrapped in edible film, the WOF in a 9-day-old treated pork patty is reduced 'down to the levels more typically found in a 3-day-old untreated' one.

Enzymes, often made using genetic modification techniques, are also creeping into our food chain to extend what the industry refers to as the 'perceived freshness' of baked goods. When we see muffins, cupcakes and soft pound cake at a coffee bar or in-store bakery, how fresh do we think they are? I'd guess that most of us would assume a couple of days old, no more. But for all we know, they have been made with an enzyme product, such as XFresh, described by its makers as follows:

> XFresh makes use of enzyme technology to prolong the sensory shelf life and perceived freshness of both pound cakes and smaller cake products like muffins, magdalenas and cupcakes. The technology has proven to be highly effective, extending the sensory shelf life by up to 50%. Consumer tests and professional panels show that applications based on XFresh technology improve the perceived freshness of cakes by up to 50%. In one instance, a four-week-old cake made with XFresh technology was judged to be as fresh as a one-week-old conventional cake.

So what if your muffin or cupcake isn't fresh from the oven? Many consumers will be only too delighted if their food keeps for longer, even if they don't know why. Few of us realise that the cosmetic perfection in chilled food we have come to expect is stage-managed. Under the coy banner of 'food protection', manufacturers now have access to various bacteria-slaying, or delaying, shelf-life extenders that are marketed as being more natural than synthetic preservatives. For instance Verdad F41, a white distilled vinegar made from sugar, corn or tapioca, was developed specifically for vacuum packed pork and poultry to help it 'maintain colour, uniformity, and reduce[s] grey discolouration during shelf life'. 'Enhanced' with this preparation, chicken thighs won't turn that off-putting yellowish-grey colour as they age. Verdad F41 is 'label friendly' – it can be described as cultured corn sugar and/or vinegar – which doesn't raise consumer hackles. But what domestic cook would 'wash' chicken in vinegar and then consider it fresh?

At the cutting edge of shelf life extension lies a new generation of preservative 'systems' or 'solutions' that combine a number of chemicals refined and isolated from food sources. Food industry chemists are busily exploring the preservative potential of oregano, rosemary, thyme, clove, cinnamon, green tea, mustard, garlic, lactic acid bacteria, lysozyme from egg white, pleurocidin from the skin of a fish, grape seeds, blueberries and cranberries. Natural preservatives already on the market include NaturFORT, promoted as 'a versatile combination of rosemary and green tea extract that complement each other by providing superior protection of flavour, colour and odour profiles' in products such as salad dressing and mayonnaise. Fortium, recommended as a shelf-life extender for crisps, is listed as a 'plant-derived product line based on mixed tocopherols and [unspecified] formulated blends' that provides 'extra protection for high stress processing conditions'. (Spuds take a bit of a pounding in the crisp factory.) BioVia™ YM 10, made from cultured dextrose and plant extracts, is marketed as a natural antifungal blend, 'specially designed to enhance the quality of a wide variety of refrigerated and shelf-stable culinary products', such as 'fresh' salsas and dips. While these preservatives can be presented as natural, what's natural about putting them in foods that would not otherwise contain them?

Arguably, these newer, 'natural' preservatives are preferable to the old synthetic ones. Do you know anyone who would like to think that their 'fresh' fish had been treated with Ecoprol 2002, a clear, light brown, slightly pungent liquid blend of propyl gallate, citric acid, potassium sorbate, orthophosphoric acid, acetic acid, and propylene glycol? The purpose of this six E number cocktail of artificial preservatives is given as follows:

> Mixture of food grade additives aimed to reduce the speed of alteration of natural marine species, allowing longer life. The antimicrobial antioxidant components act as highly effective preservative that extends the shelf life of seafood, especially in the commercialisation [sales] stage, without altering the taste, colour, odour, or texture. The additive components act to provide a protective coating against deterioration of fresh produce by microbial action, oxidation of fats and oils, and body dehydration.

In comparison to old, unreconstructed synthetic chemical concoctions such as this, any life-extending substance that bears some faint claim to naturalness represents progress. Or does it? The old arsenal of preservatives, whatever its collective impact on human health, at least did the job of preserving food, albeit in a thuggish way. Milder-mannered 'natural' alternatives are much less effective, possibly even 'a disaster waiting to happen', as one food industry chemist has warned:

> Because we have safe and reliable [synthetic] preservatives we have managed to keep products safe throughout their shelf-life. But with the demand for all-natural, minimally processed products with an extended shelf-life, the potential for low-level contamination is raised.

In other words, if you reduce the use of artificial preservatives without also shortening use-by dates, you have the recipe for a major food poisoning incident caused by chilled, supposedly fresh food.

In the past, it was blindingly obvious when food was not fresh. It stank, grew whiskers, oozed ominous liquids, discoloured, and developed warning moulds. Before the era of domestic refrigeration, we used chilly pantries to postpone for a few days this inevitable decay, and had a solid, empirical grasp of the keeping properties of foods. We relied on venerable preservation techniques – drying, curing, pickling, fermentation, brining, freezing, preservation in salt, sugar, alcohol, bottling – to extend the edible life of our food further. In time, the emerging food industry developed techniques, such as canning and ultra-heat treatment, which allowed us to eat food years after its natural 'start date'. Nevertheless, we understood that a can of peas, or dried milk powder, although still fit for consumption, wasn't exactly fresh in the fullest sense of that word. Those peas weren't from a freshly picked pod, that milk had come more recently from a factory than a cow. We knew that something had been done to these foods to make them last longer than they otherwise would. Nowadays, many of us have only the haziest idea of how long foods will keep in the natural course of events. Refrigeration has become a surrogate for genuine freshness. Anything that is cool to the touch gives us an unwarranted sense of security.

Whose fault is that? Hazy consumer awareness of the keeping potential of foods is a state of (un)consciousness that has been encouraged by food processors and retailers. Back in 1987, the food scientist Dr Robert L. Shewfelt coined the term 'fresh-like' to describe that booming category of products that seem fresh, but aren't, and this adjective has since slipped seamlessly into the lexicon of modern food processing. In the food industry, 'fresh' now means 'fresh-like', a word play that suits food manufacturers and retailers. Fresh-like foods are a money-spinner – we pay a premium for them, thinking that they are truly fresh.

What hard facts does the word 'fresh' actually convey these days? To be honest, this adjective is well-nigh meaningless.

14

Packed

Every scrap of factory-made food we eat has to be packed. Packaging protects food on its long journey from the processing plant to shops and supermarkets, and to our homes. It carries the marketing images that sell the product to us, images that frequently bear very little resemblance to the product within. One Twitter commentator posted a picture of a sad-looking pile of unidentifiable red and beige objects in a black plastic container next to the altogether more beguiling image of reduced-calorie chicken enchiladas on the covering sleeve, along with the obvious question: 'Dear @asda look at this. Do you think the food looks yummy just like the picture?' A reflection that often drifts into the minds of convenience food consumers when the reality looks about half as delectable as the lip-smacking food styling and professional photography on the box would lead one to suppose.

A vehicle for both transportation and marketing, packaging creates the heft in the contemporary shopping trolley. In the lowest grade processed food ranges, packaging often dwarfs the food in volume. Those who bother to recycle food packaging will soon notice how those cartons, containers, wrappers, films, liners, cans, bags, bottles, lids and sleeves stack up. For those who don't, the problem of excess packaging is transferred, out of sight, out of mind, to landfill dumps.

A ready-made pizza, for instance, often sits on a polystyrene disc, swathed in clingy plastic wrapping, inside a plasticised cardboard sleeve or box. When we pull off the wrapper, some of the pizza topping usually comes away with it, evidence of contact. In factory food, a number of polymer plastics hold pre-cooked ingredients in their sticky, clammy embrace, all the while exchanging body fluids. The film on ready meals that turns brittle once cooked according to the manufacturer's instructions is dotted with steamy brown liquid that drips onto the food contents in the shallow plastic tray, a humid haze of reheated industrial ingredients and hot plastic. Prawn mayonnaise sandwiches and Peking duck wraps sit in the supermarket and takeaway shop chiller for 48 hours, oozing their sweet, oily innards onto the plastic and cardboard carton, a carton that has absorbed printing ink, and is most likely laminated with an ultra-fine plastic film.

To prevent the metal reacting with the contents, tinned food languishes for years at a time inside cans lacquered with epoxy resins – better known for their use as ingredients in glue – or various plastic coatings. Raw and more minimally processed foods also get up close and personal with a gamut of advanced food packaging materials. Supermarket meat is displayed on a plastic tray upon an absorbent mat that discreetly soaks up any blood, lest the queasy consumer is reminded that this flesh was once part of an animal. Cheeses – even those with an external wrapper made of waxed paper to create the mood of an artisan cheesemonger's shop – are often clad in tight-fitting plastic underwear. Most people won't choose the more expensive oil in a glass bottle, opting instead for the usual rigid plastic container. Children go off to school with a suckable plastic yogurt tube in their lunch box, or a stiffer plastic mini-pot of fromage frais. They drink juice through a plastic straw from a cardboard container coated with a plastic polymer, and lined with metal foil. Over-priced raspberries are presented like royalty on the red carpet in a crystal-clear plastic container, under a layer of 'breathable' film, atop an absorbent crimson 'bubble pad' that disguises any juice leakage; such pads can be supplied to packers pre-treated with shelf-life extending fungicides if desired. The insides of the brown cardboard takeaway boxes used by food pop-ups and stalls at outdoor events are coated with wax, usually petroleum-based.

The range of packaging materials and substances now available to the food manufacturer is elaborate and futuristic, with innovative new concepts coming onto the market constantly. Many forms of plastic food packaging, used for products such as ready grated cheese, are often treated with a microscopic layer of chemicals, such as alkyl mono- and disulfonic acids, aluminium borate and N,N-bis(2-hydroxyethyl) dodecanamide. They provide an 'anti-fog' effect by stopping build-up of dewy moisture in the container, or act as 'anti-statics', performing a non-stick function that allows foods such as honey, chocolate sauce and grated cheese to slip more easily from the pack. If, for example, you have ever felt cheated when those last remnants of ketchup remained stubbornly at the bottom of the container, you might be receptive to cutting edge LiquiGlide; although you are unlikely to be aware of its presence because packaging substances are not listed on food labels. LiquiGlide's makers describe it as follows:

> Liquid-impregnated surfaces are a patent-pending, super-slippery surface technology that comprise a composite of solid and liquid materials, where the solid holds the liquid tightly at the surface and the liquid provides the lubricity.

Reportedly, LiquiGlide was initially invented for coating car windshields and airplane wings, but it has more recently been reformulated for food use as a product to line glass, plastic and metal packaging for foods. When applied to the inside of a bottle, the walls are so lubricated that condiments that would normally stick to the inside almost fall out. Slick is the word that sums up LiquiGlide. Mayonnaise dispensers treated with it are due to hit the shelves in 2015.

As you can see, food packaging technology is tirelessly revolutionary, with up-to-the-minute, game-changing options becoming available to food manufacturers all the time. One of the latest films, designed to pack cooked meats, cheese, milk, condiments and salad dressings, is composed of no fewer than seven microscopically thin plastic layers, and is described as follows:

> A multilayer plastic film comprising polyethylene outer layers with inner layers of additional polyethylene adjacent to tie layers of adhesive bonded to a blended polyamide and polyvinyl alcohol core. This structure results in excellent oxygen and water barrier properties. The film can be co-extruded in a blown film process that results in a durable barrier film without the sacrifice of optical properties.

Shall I run that by you once again? Unless you are an expert on polymer chemistry, this description may not mean much.

Suffice it to say, this film keeps out air and moisture, yet still looks attractive on the shelf. Most of us don't have much insight into the composition of food packaging materials, which, if they ring a bell at all, we more associate with non-food contexts, substances such as nitrocellulose, polypropylene, nylon, polyester, aluminium, polyethylene, polycarbonate and vinyl chloride are more likely to make us think of flooring, plant pots, clothing, computers, and so on.

If you mainly cook from scratch at home, this limits your exposure to such food contact materials. In the domestic setting, we tend to chop on wood, cook with steel utensils, and serve what we prepare on or in ceramic and glass, materials that have a long history of food usage. The exceptions here are non-stick pots and pans, and plastic chopping boards, both of which are controversial. In the case of non-stick, the concern is that when non-stick cookware is overheated, scratched, or even broken down at a molecular level invisible to the naked eye, a whole chemistry set of compounds come off in our food, notably fluoropolymers, not generally recommended for human consumption. And while plastic chopping boards were once promoted by food safety authorities as being more hygienic than wood, evangelical ardour for them waned when an independent study, conducted by the Food Safety Laboratory at the University of California, Davis, concluded that 'wooden cutting boards are not a hazard to human health, but plastic cutting boards may be'.

These exceptions apart, if your diet centres on real food prepared at home, food contact materials won't loom so largely in your life, although scarcely a soul will get by without using the odd roll of aluminium foil or cling film, some canned food, plastic milk bottles, and plastic sleeves inside cardboard boxes of dried foods, such as rice and breakfast cereals. Packaging is an inevitability of modern life. But heavy consumers of ready-prepared food are exposed to these materials repeatedly, on a daily basis. Over 6,000 chemicals are used to make food packaging, be it plastic, cardboard, paper, glass or metal, so whether it's the supermarket sushi, the sandwich, the salad bowl, the smoothie, the sponge cake, the salami, or the soup, the factory-made, processed food that passes through our mouths to our stomachs cohabits intimately with packaging chemicals for most of its life.

Does this matter? According to the UK's FSA, it doesn't. With the customary nonchalance displayed by this body charged with oversight of public health, it assures us that food packaging is safe and meets European standards. 'Consumers should not be concerned by the presence of chemicals in food contact materials if they are used within any limits or restrictions set for their use', it says.

So that's all right then ... or is it? The Food Packaging Forum, a not-for-profit, independent foundation that examines the science around packaging, thinks differently. It constantly reviews scientific data on which chemicals migrate from food contact materials into food and beverages, under which conditions, and at what levels, monitoring research on the human health consequences of chronic, low-dose contamination. In this capacity, it recently warned that 175 dangerous chemicals are found in food packaging, chemicals defined by international chemical classification bodies as 'Chemicals of Concern' (COCs) because they have been linked to cancer, reduced fertility, genital malformations and hormone disruption, and so may present an unreasonable risk of injury to the environment and health.

The list of toxic chemicals routinely and legally used to pack what we eat and drink is an eye-opener. To give you a flavour, it includes substances such as formaldehyde, benzene, propylparaben, ammonia, toluene, perchloroethylene, carbon monoxide, asbestos and chlorinated paraffin. These are amongst the more readily accessible, more pronounceable chemicals amongst wordier inclusions, such as 2-octyl-(4-dimethyl-amino)benzoic acid, tert-butylhydroxyanisole (BHA), 1,2,3-trichloropropane, diisodecyl phthalate (1,1,3,3-tetramethylbutyl)phenol, (2,3-Epoxypropyl)trimethyl-ammonium chloride, and 4-(1,1,3,3-tetramethylbutyl)-phenyl-polyethylene glycol nonylphenol, ethoxylated. Amidst this lengthy list of toxic substances are chemicals that have long been linked to chronic health concerns: phthalates in plasticisers; benzophenones in inks and plastic coatings; BPA in plastics and can linings; and organotin compounds in tins.

How can this be permitted? Food contact materials have long been in the frame as a possible major source of chronic exposure to chemicals, and in a horrible synergy, their toxicity can be increased in the presence of other chemicals that have the same mode of action. Packaging manufacturers are legally obliged to guarantee that their products 'do not transfer their constituents to food in quantities which could endanger human health', so who would expect that chemicals known to be toxic would be used intentionally in food contact materials? After all, many of them match the criteria for 'Substances of Very High Concern' set by REACH, the Registration, Evaluation, Authorisation and Restriction of Chemicals, the European Union's chemical authorisation body. Under European rules, chemicals that have highly toxic properties must be registered and approved for use, but the guidelines do not cover food packaging. So perversely, although REACH requirements extend to chemicals used in the making of toys, paints, textiles, medical equipment and other diverse goods, they do not cover food contact materials, even though many people are exposed to them repeatedly, every day of their lives, sometimes with each meal or snack they eat.

Why aren't packaging chemicals more controlled? Brinkmanship with potentially dangerous chemicals is hard-wired into the industrial food system. It operates on the smug assumption that known toxins have no harmful effect, provided they are at a low enough concentration, or dose. This comforting conclusion is drawn from the musings of the 16th-century Swiss physician, Paracelsus, who said: 'All things are poison, and nothing is without poison: the dose alone makes a thing not poison'. This wisdom has since been condensed into a more clubbable phrase that has since become the foundational dogma of contemporary chemical safety testing: 'The dose makes the poison'. Or, to paraphrase: a small amount of a poison does you no harm.

But when Paracelsus sat down at the table he didn't ping a chicken tikka ready meal in the microwave, or quench his thirst with soft drinks from a can. His diet wasn't composed of takeaways in polystyrene and supermarket reheats swathed in plastic. Nor was he exposed to synthetic chemicals in the environment as we are now: in traffic fumes, in pesticides, in furnishings, in fact in just about everything. If we time-travelled Paracelsus to the present day to note the ubiquity of food packaging made with chemicals that have known toxic properties, perhaps he might feel the need to update his words of wisdom. Real-world levels of exposure to toxic chemicals are not what they were during the Renaissance.

And many researchers now believe that some chemicals have unexpected and potent effects at very low doses that Paracelsus didn't anticipate. Bisphenol A (BPA) is a case in point. Used to line cans, and to make plastic containers, it is one of the most hotly contested packaging chemicals. Concluding one of the largest reviews of independent, non-industry research literature on bisphenol A, an expert panel warned:

> The wide range of adverse effects of low doses of bisphenol A in laboratory animals exposed both during development and in adulthood is a great cause for concern with regard to the potential for similar adverse effects in humans. Recent trends in human diseases relate to adverse effects observed in experimental animals exposed to low doses of BPA. Specific examples include: the increase in prostate and breast cancer, urogenital abnormalities in male babies, a decline in semen quality in men, early onset of puberty in girls, metabolic disorders including insulin resistant (type 2) diabetes and obesity, and neurobehavioral problems such as attention deficit hyperactivity disorder.

A sobering assessment, but despite such warnings, the scientific 'consensus' needed to get regulators to act on the health risks of bisphenol A is not deemed to have been established, a situation not entirely unconnected with the packaging industry's determination to quash any suggestion that its products might possibly cause harm. There are parallels here with the long war fought over proving the harm done by tobacco. Independent scientists were ringing alarm bells and regulators and consumers were acting on their advice, long before the damage caused by tobacco was 'proved' conclusively.

The same thing is happening with bisphenol A. However much the industry rebuts its critics and seeks to influence the bodies that regulate chemicals, the world is not wholly persuaded. Public concern has resulted in a ban on bisphenol A in packaging and reusable food containers, such as 'sippy cups', intended for children under the age of three in Canada, the European Union and the USA, and after a re-evaluation carried out by the French National Agency for Food, Environmental and Occupational Health and Safety, the French National Assembly and Senate voted to ban BPA from all food contact products by January 2015. Several cancer charities now advise people to avoid bisphenol A. Breast Cancer UK has called for a ban on bisphenol A in all food and drink packaging. Despite the determination of the packaging industry, the bad news about this chemical just won't go away.

Another group of packaging chemicals, phthalates, has also been under the spotlight. These plasticisers, which are added to films and other packaging materials to keep them soft, have been shown to migrate into foods, particularly fatty ones; phthalates are 'lipophilic', that is to say, they like to hang out with fat. But fatty foods are not the only type of food that might be contaminated by phthalates. The highest levels of certain phthalates have been found in bread, not a fatty food.

Now the presence of phthalates in our bread, or any other food, is worrying because tests on animals link these chemicals to reduced fertility, and reproductive and testicular toxicity. And in people, increased levels of phthalates are associated with obesity and reduced masculinisation in newborn boys.

Yet phthalates are all around us. In 2012 the UK's FSA reported that 31 per cent of foods tested contained phthalates above the level set in European law. The contaminated packaging materials in question included a glass jar metal closure with PVC, a plastic container with a foil lid, a beverage carton made of paper, foil and plastic laminate, a foil-lined pouch, and several plastic bags in carton boxes. Just the sort of thing that all of us have in our kitchens.

And what about more commercial catering? When scientists at the University of Naples examined cooked food sent from a central kitchen to nursery and primary schools in sealed disposable dishes made from packaging materials with polyethylene and polyethylene terephthalate-coated aluminium foil, nearly all of it (92 per cent) contained a phthalate. Fish and bread had the highest concentrations. This adds to the considerable body of evidence supporting the not revolutionary proposition that chemicals from packaging can leach into our food. Clearly, such exposure is not inevitable. Why not have kitchens in each school where paid people prepare fresh food on wood, steel, glass and ceramic? In this sense, the container-loads of throwaway materials that now swathe and embalm our food and drink are the packaging equivalent of the zero hours contract. They represent a disinvestment in permanency and durability, be that re-usable utensils or people, for an industrial food system that encourages disposability, a system based on short-term savings that doesn't factor in the cost to human health.

Controversy over chemicals, such as bisphenol A and phthalates, has been aired for decades, but the same cannot be said for nanoparticles, an emerging technology. Nanoparticles, which are far too minute to see with a microscope, are derived from materials such as clay, silver, titanium, silica and zinc oxide, and are increasingly used in food and drink packaging. They can perform certain 'smart' functions: extending the shelf life of food by decreasing the permeability of plastics, acting as anti-bacterial coatings, or making packaging lighter and stronger. Nanosilver, for example, is used to coat plastic food containers so that anything stored within can be sold for longer. Nanoclays can be incorporated into the fabric of plastic bottles to prevent oxygen from migrating through the walls and shortening the shelf life of the contents.

A boon for the food industry and consumers, surely? Unfortunately, in echoes of bisphenol A and phthalates, it looks as if nanoparticles can also leach from packaging into food and drink. Researchers recently found, for instance, that aluminium and silicon nanoparticles migrated from plastic bottles into an acidic medium – of the kind you find in fizzy drinks and juices – and that this migration increased with time, and at higher temperatures.

Should we be worried? The potential health problem with nanoparticles is their minuteness. They are about one ten-thousandth the width of a human hair, which makes them more reactive and more bioactive than larger particles of the same substance. This means they can end up in places that larger particles would not – our cells, tissues and organs, where they can accumulate to ill effect. Nanoscale zinc oxide, for example, has been found to cause lesions in the liver, pancreas, heart and stomach in laboratory animals. The European Commission's Scientific Committee on Consumer Safety has warned that 'clear positive toxic responses [in some of these tests] clearly indicate a potential risk [of nanoscale zinc oxide] to humans'. Other research suggests that nanoparticles of titanium dioxide can damage DNA, disrupt cell function, and interfere with the defence activities of the immune system. One emerging scientific theory is that nanoparticles absorbed in the gut may be a factor in the growing prevalence of inflammatory conditions such as irritable bowel syndrome, and Crohn's disease.

The European Commission acknowledges that nanoparticles could cause health damage. It cites evidence from laboratory studies that nanoparticles can promote clumping of protein molecules, a factor in a number of medical conditions. It also acknowledges that they can be transported from the upper lining of the nose [by inhalation] into the lungs and brain, a particular hazard for factory workers who have to handle nanomaterials. 'Full evaluation of the potential hazards is still to come', the European Commission reports, in a vaguely promising sort of way. In the USA, the National Academy of Sciences is more impatient and warns that 'critical gaps' in understanding [of nanoparticles] have been identified but 'have not been addressed with needed research'. Basically, nanotechnology is out and about, and in contact with our food and drink. Regulators have been caught on the hop. The Institute of Food Science and Technology – the professional body of food technologists – has expressed concern that nanoparticles are being used in food packaging, despite migration rates and exposure risks being unknown, and it notes:

> There does not appear to be a requirement for the supplier to specify the inclusion of nanoparticles in packaging materials and neither, due to the lack of end-product label-

> ling requirements, is the consumer likely to be aware of the composition of the packaging material.

About 400–500 nanopackaging products are estimated to be in use now, and nanotechnology is predicted to account for 25 per cent of all food packaging by 2020. In fact, packaging is just the advanced guard for this novel technology; nanotech additives are already out in force on US shelves. Nanosized titanium dioxide, for example, is now turning up in products such as coffee creamer, cookies, cream cheese, turkey gravy, lemonade and chocolate. Fresh fruit and vegetables can also be coated with a thin, wax-like coating, containing nanoparticles, to extend shelf life.

Could nanotech additives also be in the UK and European food chain? The truth is that no-one really knows, and there has been no legal obligation on food manufacturers to inform us of their presence. In Europe, the labelling of food products containing nanoparticles has been a battleground. As usual, large food manufacturers and the nanotech lobby have been lobbying for light-touch regulation that would allow them generous room for manoeuvre. A European Union regulation that requires foods (not packaging) containing nanoparticles to be labelled with the word 'nano' in brackets next to the relevant ingredient or additive came into force in December 2014. In theory, this should flag up whether the silver in your cake decorations and up-market chocolates, or the titanium dioxide in your marshmallows and icings, have a nanohistory. But don't expect the shelves to be flooded with such nanolabels. Food and drink manufacturers continue to wrangle with regulators over the exact definition of nanoparticles, arguing that they have been using the same materials for years.

Titanium dioxide in its conventional form, for instance, already has an E number: E171. It is also extremely difficult to detect and test for 'intentionally introduced' nanoparticles in food and drink, so ultimately, manufacturers risk little legal wrath if they continue to use ingredients in their nano form in products without also using the word 'nano' on the label.

So nanoparticles may very well continue to be the ultimate mystery ingredients not only in packaging, but also in food and drink. Indeed, a considerable effort is under way to push nanotechnology deep into the fabric of our food chain. Many transnational food and drink companies are investing heavily in nanotech research and development, and going by their track records, will expect a return on their investment.

The thing is, whether you're talking imperceptible nanoparticles, or the well-stocked pharmaceutical cabinet of chemicals that perform sterling service in the production of food and drink packaging, the obvious question arises – just how many minute doses of toxins can we be exposed to before our bodies abandon resistance and get ill? Toxins, just like bad luck and playground bullies, gang up, and when they do, the results aren't pretty.

Who doesn't know someone with a food allergy, or asthma, or irritable bowel syndrome, or with cancer, for that matter? Closed-minded toxicologists refer back to the philosophical musings of Paracelsus to justify an accommodating attitude to toxic compounds in our food chain and environment as they examine each one in splendid isolation from the safe confines of the laboratory. The rest of us, however, are right to question the comforting pronouncement of the imperturbable Paracelsus, frozen in the 16th century, that small doses of poison do us no harm. We can be open-minded enough to consider the very real possibility that by activating, blocking, hijacking or otherwise messing with the normal functioning of our bodies, engineered chemicals are contributing to a wide range of human health problems, including obesity, diabetes, cancer, cardiovascular disease, infertility and other disorders of sexual development. And if we do take this proposition seriously, then reducing our exposure by minimising the amount of packaged food and drink we consume is one obvious place to start.

Postscript

On the morning of 1 January 2014, I found myself standing in a blissfully quiet Rijksmuseum in Amsterdam, looking at Floris Claesz. van Dijck's inimitable painting, *Still Life with Cheese*. A table is draped in a damask cloth with a remarkably life-like meal set out upon it. Rough-hewn cheese, stacked in rugged halves, forms the centre point. Bowls spilling over with apples, pears and grapes flank the cheese. In the foreground, next to crusty bread rolls, lies a half-eaten pear on a pewter plate, some cracked nutshells, and a curling ribbon of fruit skin. A paring knife rests on the cheese plate behind a half drunk glass of wine or water, as if the person who was eating this simple yet generous meal had just left the table for a few minutes to do something else.

Van Dijck was a celebrated 'alte meister' of the Dutch Still Life school that flourished in Europe's Low Countries in the 1600s, which was renowned, amongst other things, for its meticulous depiction of food. Throughout the Netherlands and Belgium, and in many of the world's most distinguished museums, you can view paintings by van Dijck and other Old Masters, showing pomegranates, lobsters, cooked hams, quinces, steaks, fish smoked and raw, cherries, loaves, game birds, raised pies, crabs, lemons, and many other ingredients from the larder of that period.

The eerie thing about these works of art is just how real and present the food seems. Looking at *Still Life with Cheese* made me hungry. I wanted to pick away at that bunch of grapes, slice myself a wedge of cheese, and maybe tear off a chunk of the bread, before the invisible diner returned.

This painting is dated as circa 1615, but it had a potent contemporaneous effect on me. The food looked so honestly good, so wholesome in a sound, intrinsic way, that it put me in mind to visit one of Amsterdam's cheese shops, then drop by one of the greengrocer's stores that are still found in the city's high-density residential areas, to put together my own little table-top feast.

A thought hit me then on that rainy reflective day that has not left me since. Even though it was painted four centuries ago, the food so carefully reproduced by van Dijck is food that I can still strongly relate to. I can instantly understand what it is. I can visualise where it came from, how it was made, grown, farmed or fished. That familiarity sharpens my appetite.

The same cannot be said for the burgeoning portfolio of modern manufactured food products that increasingly occupy the foreground of our diets. Presented with contemporary shopping trolleys filled with elaborate edible constructions, van Dijck, his contemporaries, and followers, would experience considerable difficulty finding something they recognised as food. 'What's this then?' they might ask, as they rummaged through the low-fat spread and Coco Pops®, perplexed. And being so scrupulous in their faithful reproduction of natural detail, I could see them scoffing at the blatant disparity, so evident to the artist's eye, between the eye-grabbing visuals on the packaging, and the drab, washed-out contents. I doubt that the appearance of many modern manufactured foods would spur them to put oil to canvas. There is so little beauty in ingredients that have been designed by food technologists and industrially processed out of their natural state.

Yet the pace of food engineering innovation means that newer, more complex creations with ever more opaque modes of production are streaming onto the market every day. As I put the finishing touches to this book, a dossier for a new line of dairy proteins drops into my mailbox. Alongside a photo of a rustic-looking, golden pan loaf, the explanation reads:

> Many bakers are now turning to permeates, a rather new ingredient in the food ingredients market. Permeate is a co-product of the production of whey protein concentrate (WPC), whey protein isolate (WPI), ultrafiltered milk, milk protein concentrate (MPC), or milk protein isolate (MPI).

Permeate, apparently, 'contributes to the browning of baked goods' and produces bread that 'retains its softness for a longer period of time and extends shelf life'. How clever. But I for one would prefer that my bread was browned solely from the application of heat. I'm prepared to accept that it will stale over a natural course of time, rather than eat something that owes its existence to ingredients and technologies I am not privy to, cannot interrogate, and so can never truly understand. Am I about to hand over all control of bread, or anything else I eat, to the chemical industry's food engineers? Not without a fight.

For most of the world's history, populations around the globe have shared a common vision and understanding of food, despite their diverse cultures and geographies. From the Ancient Greeks to the Victorians, civilisations down the ages would be able to identify every ingredient in van Dijck's *Still Life with Cheese*, and the food so beautifully depicted in this painting still speaks clearly to me. But if we laid out a more contemporary artwork, let's call it *Still Life with Processed Food*, none of us, past or present, would really be any the wiser. Manufactured food relies on words to identify itself. Real food needs no explanation. It is instantly accessible to everyone, everywhere, any time.

Notes

Introduction

'You will still find it hard to avoid the 6,000 food additives': W. Kamuf *et al.*, 'Overview of caramel colours', http://www.ddwcolor.com/Caramel-Overview.pdf

'Norfolk turkey king, Bernard Matthews, abruptly terminated a face-to-face interview': Bernard Matthews obituary, *Guardian*, 26 November 2010: http://www.theguardian.com/business/2010/nov/26/bernard-matthews-obituary

'In food manufacturing, no one seems to blink at stumping up £1,999 for a conference pass, or paying £399 upwards for a workshop': Fi Global Summit 2014, https://registration.n200.com/survey/0agc7rw9lg3q9

Food Flavours & Flavour Enhancers: Market, Technical & Regulatory Insights, Leatherhead Food Research: http://www.leatherheadfood.com/food-flavours

George Orwell: *The Road to Wigan Pier*, Penguin Modern Classics, pages 91–92

'This industry is just so damn profitable.' Food and drink manufacturing is a great British success story: FDF: Ingredients For Success, https://www.fdf.org.uk/publicgeneral/Ingredients-for-success.pdf

The UK Department of Health's 'eatwell plate': http://tna.europarchive.org/20100929190231/http://www.food.gov.uk/images/pagefurniture/ewplatelargefeb10.jpg

The 'Don't Cook, Just Eat!' campaign: http://www.just-eat.co.uk/dontcook

'I feel more affinity with the message of the mysterious graffiti artist in Cologne': Graffiti Artist Defaces Fast-Food Billboards with Healthy Recipes: Delish.com, 14 November 2013: http://www.delish.com/food/recalls-reviews/graffiti-artist-defaces-fast-food-billboards-with-recipes

Chapter 1

Vesta chicken curry: www.cookdandbombd.co.uk: http://img831.imageshack.us/img831/5894/vestac.jpg

Sir Gulam Noon, 'High Noon for the ready meals industry', *Financial Times*, 8 February 2013

'Lasagne and chicken tikka are now the two best sellers': author factory visit

'By 2013, UK-based food companies were manufacturing over 12,000 different chilled food recipes': Greencore careers leaflet, http://www.greencore.com/assets/docs/CFA_Careers_Leaflet.pdf

'This is a big business – over £10 billion a year': Defra tweet c. 1 August 2013

'Which represents some 13% of the UK's total retail food market': CFA Media+Chilled bites, http://www.chilledfood.org/MEDIA/CHILLED+BITES

'Within this grand total, ready meals are by far the largest sales category': UK Chilled Food Market Report 1999–2005 (CFA)

'The UK ate its way through 3 billion of them in 2012': ITV *Tonight* Food Facts and Fiction, 16 August 2013

'Now, according to Greencore': Greencore careers leaflet, http://www.greencore.com/assets/docs/CFA_Careers_Leaflet.pdf

'As one government food safety manual puts it': A Guide to Calculating the Shelf Life of Foods, New Zealand Food Safety Authority, http://www.foodsafety.govt.nz/elibrary/industry/guide_calculating-contains_background.pdf

'The Chilled Food Association presents its industry's products as "local"': CFA Media+Chilled bites, http://www.chilledfood.org/MEDIA/CHILLED+BITES

'Food should be simple, well cooked and flavoursome': CFA website: A chef's life, http://www.chilledfood.org/MEDIA/A+chefs+life

'When on ITV *Tonight* investigation': 'Food Facts and Fiction', ITV *Tonight*, 12 August 2013

'Around 40 per cent of the chicken we eat in the UK is imported': *ibid*

'Pre-fried or grilled aubergines, peppers and courgettes': Dujardin product list

'Eggs are supplied to food manufacturers ... in powders, with added sugar': Sanovo Egg Group: whole egg powders, http://www.sanovo.com/Whole-Egg-Powders.3266.aspx

'For manufacturing products like Scotch eggs and egg mayonnaise': British Lion egginfo website, Ready Egg Products, http://www.egginfo.co.uk/egg-products

'Extended shelf life' (one month): *ibid*

'They may be liquid, concentrated, dried, crystallised, frozen, quick frozen or coagulated': CFA, Best practice guidelines for production of chilled foods

'Hardboiled, tubular eggs': Eurovo, professional product range brochure

'Egg replacers': Egg replacers' million-pound benefits, http://www.foodmanufacture.co.uk/NPD/Egg-replacers-million-pound-benefits, *Food Manufacture*, 31 October 2012

'Everything from "predust" and "adhesion"': Newlywed Foods, http://www.nwfap.com/products

'As one supplier of batters explains': http://www.newlywedsfoods.co.uk/index.php/products/batters

'Rather than making potato gnocchi from freshly boiled potatoes, flour and egg': Emflake 3890; Emsland-Stärke GmbH

'Barbecue glazes': MRC The Flava People website, http://www.mrcflava.co.uk/our-products/

'Manufacturers can achieve that just marinated look in minutes': ITV *Tonight*; 'Food Facts and Fiction', 16 August 2013

'Providing complete, tailored solutions for a wide range of applications': Synergy seasonings, http://uk.synergytaste.com/index.asp?PageID=153

'As the marketing blurb for one such company expresses it': *ibid*

'A touch of liquid ham and cheese flavouring': Unique food processing solutions, http://www.uniqueingredients.com/liquid_flavour_systems.html

'A machine that sprays on caramel': Unique food processing solutions; spray preparations, http://www.uniqueingredients.com/spraying.html

Chinese glaze ingredients: http://www.tesco.com/groceries/Product/Details/?id=271799371

Butter extract: FLAVEX Naturextrakte GmbH

Butter powder: EPI butter powder

Cream powder: EPI cream powder

Freeze-dried apricots: A&S Biotec

'Only short-term agreements': CFA Climate Change Agreement; Chilled Food Sector Progress and Barriers

Chapter 2

25 major chilled food companies: http://www.chillededucation.org/industry-info/

Defra tweet 30 July 2013: The UK's chilled prepared food industry employs 60000 inc 1000 scientists at 100+ UK sites @bisgovuk @DefraGovUK

'Although 95% of the chilled prepared foods Britain eats is sold under a retailer's brand': Chilled Food Association website, Chilled Bites, http://www.chilledfood.org/MEDIA/POSITION+STATEMENTS/Chilled+Prepared+Meals

'Sauces are cooked by the ton then spewed out onto other food components that are cooked on a conveyor belt': ITV *Tonight*, 'Food Facts and Fiction', 16 August 2013

'Ten tons of chicken tikka a day': Noon Foods; ITV *Tonight*, 'Food Facts and Fiction', 16 August 2013

'A high staff turnover and rates of sickness absence are par for the course': letter to *Guardian* from Dave Prentis, Unison, 24 July 2014, http://www.theguardian.com/world/2014/jul/24/scandal-profits-come-before-food-safety

'Many major plants are consistently understaffed and rely on agencies to fill the gaps': *ibid*

'The use of temporary agency labour is commonplace': Hovis workers begin strike at Premier Foods factory in Wigan, *The Grocer*, 28 August 2013, http://www.thegrocer.co.uk/companies/suppliers/premier-foods/hovis-workers-begin-strike-at-premier-foods-factory-in-wigan/348863.article

'A ready meals factory can be churning out 250,000 individual servings a day, made up of 60 or 70 different products, using ten different assembly lines': author factory visit

'One leading ready meals manufacturer ... boasts': Noon Foods; ITV *Tonight*, 'Food Facts and Fiction', 16 August 2013

'More than 55 per cent of all registered UK food establishments did not receive a local authority health inspection': Restore inspection across the food industry, Unite press release, 25 July 2014, http://www.politicshome.com/uk/article/102288/unite_restore_inspection_across_the_food_industry.html, http://multimedia.food.gov.uk/multimedia/pdfs/board/board-papers-2013/lafoodlaw-annual-report-1213.pdf

Julia Long, Unite: *ibid*

'Using a system known as HACCP': http://en.wikipedia.org/wiki/Hazard_analysis_and_critical_control_points

Product recalls on 25 February 2014: Sainsbury's recalls its Frozen Sticky Toffee Sponge Pudding, M&S Lightly Dusted Salt and Pepper British Chicken Fillets withdrawn, Sainsbury's Taste the Difference Roasted Chestnut, Toasted Hazelnut & Thyme Stuffing withdrawn

FSA research on nut allergy labelling: http://multimedia.food.gov.uk/multimedia/pdfs/nutallergyresearch.pdf

Tesco mouldy rice: FSA recall, http://www.food.gov.uk/news-updates/recalls-news/2013/aug/ambient#.Uw4tXP2MNSU

'2,000 portions of rice at a time': ITV *Tonight*, 'Food Facts and Fiction', 16 August 2013

Chapter 3

'E numbers have a very high "label-polluting" effect': Dr Jan van Loo of Beneo Group in 'Ingredients Insight, Natural selection: clean label and natural ingredients', 1 November 2013

'One of the problems we face is people's confidence in chemicals': Phil Hood, Consumer Engagement Centre Lead – Europe, Unilever, http://www.foodanddrinkeurope.com/Products-Marketing/Celebrity-chefs-needed-to-sell-food-science-to-consumers/?utm_source=newsletter_weekly&utm_medium=email&utm_campaign=Newsletter%2BWeekly&c=lQa1YdAlYo54tSsMPhMPBM2ahiIIgSyR, http://www.ingredients-insight.com/features/featurehealthy-trends-clean-label-and-natural-ingredients/

'With well over 2,300 additives currently approved for use': http://www.foodadditives.org/pdf/Food_Additives_Booklet.pdf

'As this industry spokesman explains': Dr Walter Lopez, Limagrain Céréales Ingrédients, http://www.lci.limagrain.com/lci/rm_10_08_11.html

Whole Foods Market 'Unacceptable Ingredients for Food': http://www.wholefoodsmarket.com/about-our-products/quality-standards/unacceptable-ingredients-food

'Many [product] formulators do turn to the list of unacceptable ingredients': Clarifying clean label, *Food Product Design*, Vol. 21 No. 5, May 2011, http://www.foodproductdesign.com/lib/download/asset-clarifying-clean-labels.ashx?item_id=4af15034-17b8-4bd4-8ea6-64a1d4dd974f

'As the director of one food market research company put it': Luisa Robertson, MMR, quoted in *Food Manufacture*, 'Clean Dream', 30 September 2013

'The clean label concept': IFi industry definition by National Starch Food Innovation 2012, http://www.cleanlabelinsights.com/Documents/IFI%20Article%20CLEAN%20LABEL%20DEFINITION%202010.pdf

Carrageenan and cancer: *Daily Mail*, 5 November 2013, Additive in everyday products 'could cause cancer', http://www.dailymail.co.uk/news/article-80857/Additive-everyday-products-cause-cancer.html

Carageenan 'is now regarded in food industry circles as an "ideally not" [to be included] additive': *Food Manufacture*, 'Clean Dream', 30 September 2013

'Explains the sales pitch for one such product': Westhove flours/Farigel; Limagrain.

Co-texturisers: Ingredion Indulge 2740, http://www.foodinnovation.com/foodinnovation/en-gb/Ingredients/CleanLabel/Pages/novation.aspx

'They bring out the more subtle differences in texture': N-Dulge, http://www.foodinnovation.com/Downloads/Company/NDULGE_brochure.pdf

Fermentation preservatives: National Marketing Institute, USA, quoted in Purac Verdad advert, *Food Product Design* magazine

Phosphate replacers: Ezimoist, Ulrick & Short, http://www.ulrickandshort.com/ezimoist.html

Rosemary extract: EFSA; Use of rosemary extracts as a food additive, http://www.efsa.europa.eu/en/efsajournal/doc/721.pdf

'Kinetic study of pilot-scale supercritical carbon dioxide extraction of rosemary (*Rosmarinus officinalis*) leaves', Mónica R. García-Risco, Elvis J. Hernández, Gonzalo Vicente, Tiziana Fornari*, Francisco J. Señoráns and Guillermo Reglero, Universidad Autónoma de Madrid, 28049 Cantoblanco, Madrid, Spain.

Carrot extract: FLAVEX Naturextrakte GmbH

Carrot extract hues, such as 'warm orange' or 'shining yellow': Doehler, Crystal Clear colours

Extracts with additives in the mix: Univar, Colours for food brochure, http://www.univarcolour.com/downloads/Univar%20Colours%20for%20Food%20Brochure.pdf

Micronised powders as colourings: A+S Biotec Nature in new dimensions, http://www.as-biotec.com/uploads/media/Lebensmittel_brosch_0413_en3_net.pdf

Burnt sugars: Aromsa, burnt caramelised sugars

'As one supplier [of caramelised sugar syrup] explains': Sethness CS5 Caramelised Sugar Syrup

Rice extract and concentrate: Ribus, http://ribus.com/company-history-our-story

'The cost saving is immediate': Ribus natural functional ingredients brochure

Yeast extracts: DSM Maxavor All Natural, http://www.dsm.com/markets/foodandbeverages/en_US/markets-home/market-savory-lp/market-savory-simplified-labels.html http://www.dsm-apps.com/savorytool_eu/index.html

Label-friendly solutions: Corbion, Purac, http://www.purac.com/EN/Food/Brands/Verdad.aspx

'Ingredients that give the impression': Dr Jan van Loo of Beneo Group in *Ingredients Insight*, 'Natural selection: clean label and natural ingredients', 1 November 2013, http://www.ingredients-insight.com/features/featurehealthy-trends-clean-label-and-natural-ingredients/

Chapter 4

Food Ingredients Europe: Who visits? http://www.foodingredientsglobal.com/europe/exhibit/who-visits

Glucono-Delta-Lactone: Roquette, Effective acidification in white cheese leaflet

Potato protein isolate: Solanic free from solutions brochure

DKSH: DKSH Performance Materials brochure

Omya: Omya Product Portfolio brochure

Helm AG: Helm AG Competence in human nutrition

Butter Buds®: Making the most of Mother Nature brochure

All in All: company leaflet

Goat flavour cheese powder: Dairygold, cheese and dairy flavours leaflet

Caramelised onion extract: DDW, caramelised fruits and vegetables

R2 Group: product brochure

Anti-foaming agents: Wacker; Silfoam/Silfar brochure

Microlys: Culinar brochure

Pulpiz™: http://www.tateandlyle.presscentre.com/Press-releases/Pulp-Performance-Tate-Lyle-Launches-PULPIZ-Pulp-Extender-Delivers-Key-Replacement-Advantages-in-43f.aspx

Oil-dispersible technology: DDW brochure, https://youtube.googleapis.com/v/5rxTYO_78vc%26hl=en_US%26start=36%26end=55

Carfosel®: Prayon, Phosphates on a plate brochure

Dairy essence: Flaverco, Cream and milk essence brochure

Scelta Mushrooms®: http://www.sceltamushrooms.com/salt-reduction#sthash.b2jDFt9b.dpuf

Dohler red brilliance: Dohler brochure, The shining spectrum of new red tones from a 100% natural source, http://www.doehler.com/en/landingpages/colours.html

Hydro-Fi™: Fiberstar, Hydro-Fi™ information leaflet

SuperStab™: Nexira product information leaflet

Bionis®: Biorigin brochure: Art in natural ingredients

Culinar Keep: Culinar brochure

Meatshure®: Balchem encapsulates brochure

Cavamax®: Wacker Life Science – Food brochure

Volactose: Volac brochure, Volactose whey permeate

NatureSeal: Agricoat, NatureSeal brochure

Chapter 5

'By the chain's own admission': Jason Danciger, Head of Hospitality & Counters, M&S Bakery, Deli, Cafe & Eateries – Jason Danciger, www.fdin.org.uk/.../Global%20Food%20.../M&S%20Bakery,%20Deli,%...

'The point of all this effort is to 'create theatre' in the food hall': *ibid*

'Profitability has tripled': *ibid*

'I then asked the M&S press centre': email to author from Laura Watt, 9 October 2013

'Real Bread Campaign ... described such in-store bakeries as "tanning salons"': http://www.dailymail.co.uk/news/article-1261107/Supermarket-bakeries-just-loaf-tanning-salons.html

Real Bread Campaign: 'Great British Fake-Off': http://www.youtube.com/watch?v=-5xsRomUdM8

'The latter additive is derived': EFSA opinion on reevaluation of mixed carotenes (E 160a (i)) and beta-carotene (E 160a (ii))

as a food additive, http://www.efsa.europa.eu/en/efsajournal/pub/2593.htm

'From wheat to eat': Greggs customer leaflet, picked up in store 8 October 2013

'Man snacks': Emine Saner, *Guardian*, 11 August 2010

I received this response from the senior manager handling the Greggs account: email from Paul Hadfield, Havas PR UK, 31 October 2013

Chapter 6

'Sugar ... is the new tobacco': *Daily Mail*, 9 January 2014, http://www.dailymail.co.uk/health/article-2536180/Sugar-new-tobacco-Health-chiefs-tell-food-giants-slash-levels-third.html

The Good Hearted Glasgow Diet Sheet: author copy, acquired 14 April 2014

Pure, White, and Deadly: How Sugar Is Killing Us and What We Can Do to Stop It, John Yudkin, 1972

Coca-Cola sponsorship of 2012 Olympic Games: http://www.coca-cola.co.uk/faq/olympic-games/why-does-coca-cola-sponsor-the-olympic-games.html

A.G. Barr sponsorship of 2014 Commonwealth Games: 'AG Barr launches £12m marketing campaign in run-up to Glasgow 2014 Commonwealth Games', *Talking Retail*, 16 January 2014, http://www.talkingretail.com/products-news/soft-drinks/ag-barr-launches-12m-marketing-campaign-in-run-up-to-glasgow-2014-commonwealth-games/

'Glasgow is the city with the lowest life expectancy in the UK': Games host Glasgow shown to have worst life expectancy in UK, *Guardian*, 16 April 2014 http://www.theguardian.com/uk-news/2014/apr/16/games-host-glasgow-worst-life-expectancy-uk

'(Scotland) ... has the worst health record in Europe': Scottish mortality rate 'among highest in Western Europe', BBC

News, 20 November 2012, http://www.bbc.co.uk/news/uk-scotland-20402129

'[The sugar lobby] effectively silenced critics': How Big Sugar muzzles journalists [author blog], http://www.joannablythmanwriting.com/Joanna_Blythman_Writing/Blog/Entries/2012/3/5_How_Big_Sugar_muzzles_journalists.html, http://www.theguardian.com/society/2013/mar/20/sugar-deadly-obesity-epidemic

'In the words of one *British Medical Journal* editorial': How science is going sour on sugar, BMJ 2013; 346: f307, http://dx.doi.org/10.1136/bmj.f307 http://www.bmj.com/content/346/bmj.f307?etoc

Fat Chance, Dr Robert Lustig, London: Fourth Estate, 2014

Nature article: 'Public health: The toxic truth about sugar', Robert H. Lustig, Laura A. Schmidt, Claire D. Brindis, Nature 482, 27–29 (02 February 2012) doi:10.1038/482027a

WHO draft guidance on sugar: WHO: Daily sugar intake 'should be halved', BBC News, 5 March 2014, http://www.bbc.co.uk/news/health-26449497

'Major refiner, AB Sugar, complained loudly': Misleading to single out sugar as lead cause of obesity, says AB sugar, *Food Navigator*, 10 February 2014, http://www.foodnavigator.com/Market-Trends/Misleading-to-single-out-sugar-as-a-lead-cause-of-obesity-says-AB-Sugar

CAOBISCO response to WHO draft guidance: CAOBISCO pleads for further scientific substantiation, 7 April 2014, http://caobisco.eu/public/images/actualite/caobisco-07042014150238-CAOBISCO-response-WHO-consultation.pdf

'The founder of one baby food company wrote passionately ...': Paul Lindley of Ella's Kitchen: Sugar witch hunt is simplistic and infantile, *The Grocer*, 14 March 2014, http://m.thegrocer.co.uk/opinion/letters/sugar-witchhunt-is-simplistic-and-infantile/355424.article

Terry Jones, the director of the Food and Drink Federation: There's too much alarm over sugar and sweeteners, *The Grocer*, 12 April 2014

Waitrose and sugar reduction: Fruit juice the target in Waitrose war on sugar, *The Grocer*, 5 April 2014

'A 100 gram, one-person can of cola contains up to nine teaspoons of sugar': White Paper Proposed Sugar Tax, Leatherhead Food Research, January 2014, http://www.leatherheadfood.com/whitepapers

'Around ten teaspoons of sugar in a meal for one': Shocking levels of sugar in UK ready meals, says *Which?*, Food and Drink Europe, 26 May 2014, http://www.foodanddrinkeurope.com/Products-Marketing/Shocking-levels-of-sugar-in-UK-ready-meals-says-Which/?utm_source=newsletter_weekly&utm_medium=email&utm_campaign=Newsletter%2BWeekly&c=lQa1YdAlY07B9CCCAN2OIAz5y8LM7FUh

'Sugar provides bulk, textural elements, browning, caramelisation and other necessary functional elements': Navigating the Landscape of Sweetener Formulations, Food Tech Toolbox, February 2014, http://toolbox.foodproductdesign.com/reports/2014/02/sweetener-formulations.aspx

'Some scientists argue that its effect [fructose] is even worse': 'Controversy: Is high fructose corn syrup worse than sugar?', *Family Doctor Magazine*, January 2009, http://www.familydoctormag.com/nutrition/1283-hfcs-the-controversy.html

HFCS is cheaper than sugar: Sugar vs. corn syrup: Sweeteners at center of bitter food fight, Fox News, 6 September 2012, http://www.foxnews.com/health/2012/09/06/sugar-vs-corn-syrup-sweeteners-at-center-bitter-food-fight/

'Consumption of this sweetener [HFCS] has been linked to gout, hypertension, fatty liver disease, type 2 diabetes, and obesity': 'Fructose-containing sugars, blood pressure, and cardiometabolic risk: a critical review', NCBI *Curr Hypertens Rep.*

2013 Aug;15(4):281–97, doi: 10.1007/s11906-013-0364-1, http://www.ncbi.nlm.nih.gov/pubmed/23793849

'This [bad] publicity has led to a subsequent set of misperceptions': 'Worried about HFCS? The "problems" have more bark than bite', *Corn Refiners Report*, 20 June 2011, https://vts.inxpo.com/scripts/Server.nxp?LASCmd=L:0&AI=1&ShowKey=5199&LoginType=0&InitialDisplay=1&ClientBrowser=0&DisplayItem=NULL&LangLocaleID=0

'The US Food and Drug Administration rejected the name change': Response to Petition from Corn Refiners Association to Authorize 'Corn Sugar' as an Alternate Common or Usual Name for High Fructose Corn Syrup, http://www.fda.gov/aboutFDA/CentersOffices/OfficeofFoods/CFSAN/CFSANFOIAElectronicReadingRoom/ucm305226.htm

'Evaporated cane juice': Draft Guidance for Industry on Ingredients Declared as Evaporated Cane Juice; Reopening of Comment Period; Request for Comments, Data, and Information; Federal Register Notice, 5 March 2014, https://www.federalregister.gov/articles/2014/03/05/2014-04802/draft-guidance-for-industry-on-ingredients-declared-as-evaporated-cane-juice-reopening-of-comment

'One such case, against leading yogurt manufacturer Chobani': 'Chobani (finally) prevails in evaporated cane juice lawsuit, but other firms still being targeted', *Food Navigator*, 27 February 2014, http://www.foodnavigator-usa.com/Regulation/Chobani-finally-prevails-in-evaporated-cane-juice-lawsuit-but-other-firms-still-being-targeted

Sweetness levels of artificial sweeteners: 'Navigating the Landscape of Sweetener Formulations', *Food Tech Toolbox*, February 2014, http://toolbox.foodproductdesign.com/reports/2014/02/sweetener-formulations.aspx

Advantame: New sweetener Advantame approved for use in EU, Food Manufacture, 4 June 2014, http://www.foodmanufacture.co.uk/Ingredients/New-sweetener-approved-for-use-Europe

'Safe for human consumption at current levels of exposure': European Food Safety Authority (EFSA), Aspartame is safe for general population, *European Health Alliance*, 12 January 2014, http://www.epha.org/a/5904

'Whole Foods Market's "black list" of unacceptable ingredients': http://www.wholefoodsmarket.com/about-our-products/quality-standards/unacceptable-ingredients-food

'Plain old sugar ... the ideal bell curve flavour profile': 'How should the industry tackle sugar reduction?' Bakery and Snacks.com, 28 March 2014, http://www.bakeryandsnacks.com/Markets/How-should-the-industry-tackle-sugar-reduction/?utm_source=newsletter_daily&utm_medium=email&utm_campaign=Newsletter%2BDaily&c=lQa1YdAlY05%2Bz08JkJrvY743ET4voNj3

'Several large-scale studies have found a positive correlation between artificial sweetener use and weight gain': 'Gain weight by "going on a diet?" Artificial sweeteners and the neurobiology of sugar cravings', Qing Yang; *Neuroscience: Yale J Biol Med*, Jun 2010; 83(2): 101–108, http://www.ncbi.nlm.nih.gov/pmc/articles/PMC2892765/

'Rats consuming artificial sweetener gained weight faster than those eating the sugar': 'A Role for Sweet Taste: Calorie Predictive Relations in Energy Regulation by Rats', Susan E. Swithers and Terry L. Davidson; *Behavioral Neuroscience* 2008, Vol. 122, No. 1, 161–173, http://www.starling-fitness.com/wp-content/uploads/bne-feb08-swithers.pdf

'A wide-ranging review of studies looking at the impact of artificial sweeteners': 'Artificial sweeteners produce the counterintuitive effect of inducing metabolic derangements', Swithers SE; *Trends Endocrinol Metab* 2013 Sep;24(9):431–41, doi: 10.1016/j.tem.2013.05.005. Epub 2013 Jul 10 http://www.ncbi.nlm.nih.gov/pubmed/23850261

'Consumption of artificially and sugar-sweetened beverages and incident type 2 diabetes', Guy Fagherazzi *et al.*; doi: 10.3945/ajcn.112.050997 *Am J Clin Nutr*, March 2013 ajcn.050997, http://

ajcn.nutrition.org/content/early/2013/01/30/ajcn.112.050997.abstract

Sweetness decoupled from caloric content offers partial, but not complete, activation of the food reward pathways: 'Gain weight by "going on a diet?" Artificial sweeteners and the neurobiology of sugar cravings', Qing Yang; *Neuroscience: Yale J Biol Med*, Jun 2010; 83(2): 101–108, http://www.ncbi.nlm.nih.gov/pmc/articles/PMC2892765/

'Another theory is that artificial sweeteners wreak havoc with our appetite-regulating hormones': Artificial Sweeteners; Also Known as Industrial Chemicals, http://www.health-choices-for-life.com/artificial_sweeteners.html

'Agave syrup ... is about one and a half times sweeter than sugar': Natural sweeteners for label appeal: Sweeteners For the Future Food Product Design, March 2012, http://www.foodproductdesign.com/lib/download.ashx?d=1645

'The Aztecs prized the agave': All about agave; What is agave nectar?, http://www.allaboutagave.com

'Agave nectar is often labelled as raw, but it is actually extracted ...': *ibid*

'Agave syrup has a higher fructose content than HFCS': 'Sugar substitutes: What's safe, and what's not', Mercola.com, 7 October 2013, http://articles.mercola.com/sites/articles/archive/2013/10/07/sugar-substitutes.aspx

'Most agave nectar or agave syrup is nothing more than a laboratory-generated super-condensed fructose syrup': *ibid*

Coca-Cola and stevia: What is Stevia/Truvia®? http://www.coca-cola.co.uk/faq/ingredients/what-is-stevia.html

'The dried leaves of stevia are ... 40 times sweeter than sugar': Stevia; Sweet but innocent, http://www.exoptron.com/stevia-sweet-but-innocent/

Truvia®: The Scoop on Truvia® Natural Sweetener, http://truvia.com/FAQ

Erythritol and flavourings in Truvia®: From nature, for sweetness, http://truvia.com/about

'One such action claimed that "reb-A is not the natural crude preparation of stevia"': Denise Howerton, US District Court/ Hawaii, 8 July 2013, https://www.truthinadvertising.org/ wp-content/uploads/2013/07/Howerton-v.-Cargill-Inc. pdf

'Sales of Sprite nosedived after stevia was added to the recipe': Sprite sales suffer slump following reduction in sugar, *The Grocer*, 26 April 2014

'The aftertaste [of stevia] was strong and unpleasant': Adam Leyland, editor of The Grocer, *ibid*

'Scientists are isolating more minor glycosides from stevia': 'The quest for a natural sugar substitute', *New York Times*, 1 January 2014, http://www.nytimes.com/2014/01/05/magazine/the-quest-for-a-natural-sugar-substitute.html?_r=0

'They [sugar alcohols] can also cause fermentation in the lower gut': Technology and ingredients to assist with the reduction of sugar; FHIS Campden BRI, January 2013, http://www.foodhealthinnovation.com/media/6741/industry_position_papers_-_technologies_to_reduce_sugar.pdf

'Natural sweeteners like those based on stevia and monk fruit ... may not have such an easy ride further down the line': Simone Baroke, 'Navigating Consumer Activism', *Boardroom Journal*, March 2014, http://www.foodproductdesign.com/ journals/2014/02/navigating-consumer-activism.aspx

'An integration of polyols, nutritive [calorie-containing] sweeteners, high-intensity sweeteners and flavours': Kathryn Deibler in 'Natural sweeteners for label appeal: Sweeteners For the Future Food Product Design', March 2012, http://www.foodproductdesign.com/lib/download.ashx?d=1645

'Strong correlation between a person's customary intake of a flavour and his or her preferred intensity for that flavour': 'Gain weight by "going on a diet?" Artificial sweeteners and the neurobiology of sugar cravings', Qing Yang; *Neuroscience: Yale J Biol*

Med, Jun 2010; 83(2): 101–108, http://www.ncbi.nlm.nih.gov/pmc/articles/PMC2892765/

Chapter 7

Fat composition of various oils: http://chartsbin.com/view/1961

Dr Serge Renaud: *Telegraph* obituary, October 2012, http://www.telegraph.co.uk/news/obituaries/9766180/Serge-Renaud.html

'As one oil company executive explains': Gerald McNeil, vice president R&D, Loders Croklaan USA, *Food Product Design*, Vol. 22, no 7, July 2012

History of trans fats: American Heart Association, a history of trans fats, http://www.heart.org/HEARTORG/GettingHealthy/FatsAndOils/Fats101/A-History-of-Trans-Fat_UCM_301463_Article.jsp, http://childhood-nutrition.com/solutions/reduce-fat/

'As one Scottish fish and chip shop owner recalls': Stefano Vella of Pizza Amore, *Fry Magazine*, 22 October 2012, http://www.frymagazine.com/news/post.php?s=2012-10-22-regional-differences&cf=oils-features

Products that still contain trans fats: Bunge, Product Solutions Information, http://www.bungebiic.com/bakery-applications-lab/downloads/BUNGE-NH-Product-Solutions.pdf

'When polyunsaturated oil degrades ... develops a distinctive taste and aroma': John Radcliffe, 'Checking the oil for snacks', *Food Product Design*, Vol 13, No10, October 2009

'As this chemical company advice service explains': Cindy Hazen, 'New Generation of Fried Foods', *Food Product Design*, Vol. 22, No. 7, July 2012

Polymers and frying: Omega-9 oils, Dow AgroSciences, http://www.omega-9oils.com/omega-9-advantage/proven-performance/get-rid-of-gunk.htm

Toxicity of aldehydes in cooking oil: Aldehydes contained in edible oils, *Food Chemistry* 2012, 131(3): 915-926, http://www.

deepdyve.com/lp/elsevier/aldehydes-contained-in-edible-oils-of-a-very-different-nature-after-dgdqUmr004

Omega-9 oils: http://www.omega-9oils.com/omega-9-advantage/healthier-profile/

Acrolein: DGF recommendations for using frying oils and fats, http://www.dgfett.de/material/recomm.php, http://www.ncbi.nlm.nih.gov/pubmed/21994168

Oxidised monomeric triglycerides: http://www.dgfett.de/material/recomm.php

'Oils are used ... for anything from 7 up to 12 days': Bill McCulloch, 'Bunge oils in Food Product Design', *Healthier Fried Foods*, Vol. 20, No. 12, December 2010

'It's a wonder that oils survive at all': Cindy Hazen, 'New Generation of Fried Foods', *Food Product Design*, Vol. 22, No. 7, July 2012

'These higher smoke-point [high oleic acid] oils extend use of frying oil': Linda Funk, executive director of the Soyfoods Council, http://www.preparedfoods.com/articles/111863-the-crunch-on-batters-and-breadings

RBD oils: Edible oil processing, AOCS Lipid Library, http://lipidlibrary.aocs.org/processing/process.html

Oil improving additives: Optimising baking and frying process using oil improving agents, Dr Christian Gertz CUH, http://www.dgfett.de/meetings/archiv/hagen2004/vortraege/gertz.pdf

'BHA "is reasonably anticipated to be a human carcinogen": *Report on carcinogens*, 12th edition 2011, http://ntp.niehs.nih.gov/ntp/roc/twelfth/profiles/ButylatedHydroxyanisole.pdf

'It remains colourless even when heated at 194°C': Camlin Fine Sciences, http://www.camlinfs.com/products.html#antoxbha

'Another long-life frying medium ... is EE': 'Mechanical oil expression from extruded soy bean samples': P.C. Bargalea, R.J. Ford *et al.*; Paper no. J8846 in *JAOCS* 76, 223–229 (February 1999)

'We had been changing our frying oil': 'The mystery of longer life frying oil'; *inform*, February 2005, Volume 16 (2), http://aocs.files.cms-plus.com/inform/2005/2/p69-72.pdf

'The process creates a contaminant, 3-MCPD': EFSA *Journal* 2013 11(9):3381 [45 pp.], doi:10.2903/j.efsa.2013.3381, http://www.efsa.europa.eu/en/efsajournal/pub/3381.html

'The European Food Safety Authority eventually concluded that acrylamide poses a bigger cancer risk to humans': 'Acrylamide is a bigger cancer risk', says EFSA, *Food Manufacture*, 1 July 2014, http://mobile.foodmanufacture.co.uk/Food-Safety/Acrylamide-in-food-could-be-bigger-cancer-risk#.U8aCjlYsrwI

'Bradford-based researchers': The Heatox Project, press release, 26 November 2007, http://www.slv.se/upload/heatox/documents/Pressrelease_HEATOX_project_completed_–_brings_new_pieces_to_the_Acrylamide_Puzzle.pdf, http://www.highbeam.com/doc/1G1-332379721.html, http://www.dailymail.co.uk/health/article-2221601/Could-eating-burnt-toast-stunt-unborn-babys-growth.html#ixzz2sqKbApHB

'To do this job, they can turn to ... sugar-based "gelators"': 'Semi-solidifying vegetable oils', *Prepared Foods*, 28 January 2014, http://www.preparedfoods.com/articles/113668-semisolidifying-vegetable-oils

NHS butter/spreads advice: NHS Live Well, dairy foods, http://www.nhs.uk/Livewell/Goodfood/Pages/milk-dairy-foods.aspx

NHS trans fats advice: NHS Live Well, What are trans fats? http://www.nhs.uk/chq/pages/2145.aspx

'The leading "heart healthy" margarine contained 21% trans fats': 'Bad advice at fault for heart disease deaths', *Guardian*, 15 April 2014, http://www.theguardian.com/society/2014/apr/15/bad-advice-heart-disease-deaths

'A major review of 21 scientific studies on fat': *Am J Clin Nutr*, 2010 Mar;91(3):535-46, doi: 10.3945/ajcn.2009.27725 Meta-analysis of prospective cohort studies evaluating the association of saturated fat with cardiovascular disease Siri-Tarino PW, Sun Q, Hu FB, Krauss RM: http://www.ncbi.nlm.nih.gov/pubmed/20071648

Study funded by British Heart Foundation: 'Association of Dietary, Circulating, and Supplement Fatty Acids With Coronary Risk: A Systematic Review and Meta-analysis', Rajiv Chowdhury *et al.*, *Ann Intern Med*, 2014; 160(6):398-406-406, doi: 10.7326/M13-1788

'Whether inter-esterified oils are any less lethal in health terms': 'Replacing trans fat: the argument for palm oil with a cautionary note on interesterification', *J Am Coll Nutr*, 2010 Jun;29(3 Suppl):253S-284S, http://www.ncbi.nlm.nih.gov/pubmed/20823487

Chapter 8

Carotex: Carotex flavours brochure

Flaverco: Flaverco cream and milk essence brochure

'Masking Stevia, potassium chloride and vitamins': *Food Business News*, 24 January 2011, http://www.foodbusinessnews.net/News/News%20Home/Features/2011/1/Masking%20off%20flavors.aspx?AdKeyword=2014RA_0121&cck=1

'Butter Buds®: Making the most of mother Nature' brochure

Masking tastes: http://www.symriseflavors.com/Symrise_Consumer_Health.pdf

Symrise: Customised masking solutions for tastes you want to hide, http://info.symriseflavors.com/MaskingBannerA.html

Kalsec: http://www.kalsec.com/files/misc/Kalsec-Flavor-Brochure.pdf

'As one flavour chemist summarises': Chris Williams, chief flavorist, WILD Flavors; *Food Product Design*, Vol. 20, No. 3, March 2010

Comax flavour solutions: http://www.comaxflavors.com/flavorlab

Examples of flavourings available: R2 Ingredients Food Ingredients brochure, Carotex flavours brochure, Comex Flavour Lab http://www.comaxflavors.com/flavorlab, Flavex http://www.flavex.co.uk/bakery, Gold Coast Flavours listing http://www.goldcoastinc.com/flavors/, Kalsec

Grill flavours: Red Arrow grill flavours, http://www.uniqueingredients.com/ra_grills.html

Tartiflette flavouring: Innovadex 410084 Saveur: http://www.innovadex.fr/Food/Detail/5513/201985/TARTIFLETTE-REF-410084

FlavorFacts: http://www.flavorfacts.org/glossary-of-terms/

2,500 approved flavouring substances: http://europa.eu/rapid/press-release_IP-12-1045_en.htm

EU approved flavouring substances list: http://eur-lex.europa.eu/LexUriServ/LexUriServ.do?uri=OJ:L:2012:267:0001:0161:EN:PDF

50 chemicals in milkshake: *Daily Mirror*, 25 April 2006; 59 ingredients in strawberry milk shake, http://www.mirror.co.uk/news/uk-news/59-ingredients-in-strawberry-milkshake-622350#ixzz2r0BF3rS4

Tastant: Medilexicon http://www.medilexicon.com/medicaldictionary.php?t=89750

'We can get compounds.': Luis Jimenez-Maroto, Sensory Coordinator, Wisconsin Center for Dairy Research, *Food Product Design*, Vol. 21, No. 11, November 2011

Dimethyl sulfide etc.: *ibid*

10,000 flavours in nature: European Flavour Association, 'Discover the world of flavours', http://www.effa.eu/en/flavours/discover-the-world-of-flavours

Flavour notes of berry, citrus and even jasmine: *Food Product Design*, Vol. 21, No. 5, March 2011

Chemicals in chocolate: Counet C.; Callemien, D.; Ouwerx C.; Collin S. (2002), 'Use of Gas Chromatography–Olfactometry To Identify Key Odorant Compounds in Dark Chocolate', *Journal of Agricultural and Food Chemistry*, Vol. 50

'Withstand whatever process it faces': Steve Wolf, director of flavor applications, Robertet Flavors, *Food Product Design*, Vol. 21, No. 5, March 2011

Difference between natural and artificial: http://www.flavorfacts.org/faqs/

Ethyl vanillin: *ibid*; *Technology Review* 17th June 2013 Green Chemists synthesise vanillin from sawdust http://www.technologyreview.com/view/516116/green-chemists-synthesise-vanillin-from-sawdust/

FTNF, FTNS, WONF: http://www.flavorfacts.org/faqs/

'Mature cheese flavourings and enzymes': *Food Product Design*, 1 February 2004, http://www.foodproductdesign.com/articles/2004/02/food-product-design-ingredient-insight-february.aspx

Solvents: processes permitted: Regulation (EC) No 1334/2008, http://eur-lex.europa.eu/LexUriServ/LexUriServ.do?uri=OJ:L:2008:354:0034:0050:en:PDF; Council Directive (88/344/EEC), http://eur-lex.europa.eu/LexUriServ/LexUriServ.do?uri=CONSLEG:1988L0344:19971223:EN:PDF

CDC and flavouring-related lung disease: http://www.cdc.gov/niosh/topics/flavorings/exposure.html

CDC NIOSH alert, Preventing lung disease in workers, http://www.cdc.gov/niosh/docs/2004-110/pdfs/2004-110.pdf

Ritter v Stiftung Warentest: http://www.reuters.com/article/2014/01/13/odd-germany-chocolate-idUSL6N0KN30920140113; http://www.confectionerynews.com/Regulation-Safety/Ritter-Sport-wins-natural-flavor-German-court-battle

EFFA and flavour preparations: http://www.effa.eu/en/flavours/discover-the-world-of-flavours

Misleading us on flavours: REGULATION (EC) No 1334/2008, section 7, http://eur-lex.europa.eu/LexUriServ/LexUriServ.do?uri=OJ:L:2008:354:0034:0050:en:PDF

Chapter 9

'The FSA explains how this sleight of hand works': *Guidelines on approaches to the replacement of Tartrazine, Allura Red, Ponceau 4R, Quinoline Yellow, Sunset Yellow and Carmoisine in food and beverages*, available at: http://www.food.gov.uk/sites/default/files/multimedia/pdfs/publication/guidelinessotonsixcolours.pdf

Professor Brian Wansink: 'The Influence of Assortment Structure on Perceived Variety and Consumption Quantities', *Science Daily*, 1 May 2004, http://www.sciencedaily.com/releases/2004/05/040511040654.html

'Colourings in surimi: Natural calcium carbonate: a multifunctional ingredient in surimi seafood', Omya product brochure

The 'Southampton Six': *Lancet*, http://www.ncbi.nlm.nih.gov/pubmed/17825405

EFSA evaluates Southampton study, http://www.efsa.europa.eu/en/press/news/ans080314.htm; BBC News, 25 May 2004, http://news.bbc.co.uk/1/hi/health/3742423.stm

FSA response to Southampton Six study: University of Southampton news release, 14 March 2008, http://www.southampton.ac.uk/mediacentre/news/2008/apr/08_65.shtml

'As one flavour company executive put it': Roee Nir, Global Commercial Manager of Lycored, quoted in *Food Processing*, May 2013

Asda cherryade and Tizer: *Guidelines on approaches to the replacement of Tartrazine, Allura Red, Ponceau 4R, Quinoline Yellow, Sunset Yellow and Carmoisine in food and beverages*, available at: http://www.food.gov.uk/sites/default/files/multimedia/pdfs/publication/guidelinessotonsixcolours.pdf

Tandoori paste: *ibid*

'By 2011, global sales of 'natural' colours were outstripping artificial ones': *Food Processing*, May 2013

'M&S ... boasts that 99% of its food is free from artificial colours: https://plana.marksandspencer.com/media/pdf/we_are_doing/health/health_progress.pdf

EUTECA: http://www.euteca.org/html/caramel.html

Formulation of caramel colourings: JEKFA: Caramel colourings, http://www.fao.org/ag/agn/jecfa-additives/specs/monograph11/additive-102-m11.pdf

Establishing safety of caramel colouring: Overview of caramel colours; Kamuf, Nixon, Parker, Barnum, Williamson, http://www.ddwcolor.com/Caramel-Overview.pdf

'In the USA, cola brands have reformulated their drinks': Coke, Pepsi to change caramel coloring recipes, Fox News, 9 March 2012, http://www.foxnews.com/health/2012/03/09/coke-pepsi-to-change-caramel-coloring-recipes/

'Described by one colour company executive as "very cheap and very white"': Lionel Schmitt, Vice President of Commercial Development, Chr Hansen Food Navigator, 19 September 2009, http://www.foodnavigator.com/Financial-Industry/Chr-Hansen-makes-natural-white-for-confectionery

'Beneo ... was heavily promoting its alternative to titanium dioxide': 'Ditch possibly carcinogenic white color', *Confectionery News*, 21 January 2013, http://www.confectionerynews.com/Ingredients/Ditch-possibly-carcinogenic-white-color-for-clean-label-rice-starch-says-Beneo

'There is no legal distinction in the European Union between synthetic colours and natural ones': *Guidelines on approaches to the replacement of Tartrazine, Allura Red, Ponceau 4R, Quinoline Yellow, Sunset Yellow and Carmoisine in food and beverages*, available at: http://www.food.gov.uk/sites/default/files/multimedia/pdfs/publication/guidelinessotonsixcolours.pdf

'There is no clear definition of what constitutes a natural food colourant': Hawkins Watts; *Natural colour*, http://www.hawkinswatts.com/prod_cols_nat.htm

NatCol definition of natural: NATCOL Position on the Term 'Natural Colour' and the Categorisation of Food Colours, http://www.natcol.org/sites/default/files/Updated%20NATCOL%20Position%20Paper%20on%20Natural%20Colours%20Final.pdf

Process for making paprika extract: EU Regulation No. 231/2012, 9 March 2012, laying down specifications for food additives, http://

eur-lex.europa.eu/LexUriServ/LexUriServ.do?uri=OJ:L:2012:083:FULL:EN:PDF

'The websites and marketing materials of colouring companies are a riot of throbbing, glowing colorants': EP Colour Dr Anthocyanins

'As the Roha colour company warns': Roha; Color Q&As, http://www.roha.com/faqs.html

Sensient: Colour book, http://www.sensient-fce.com/fileadmin/pdf/SFC-01013_Colour_Book_PDF_RL02.pdf

Hawkins Watts: Pantone colour chart, http://www.hawkinswatts.com/toolbox-pantonechart.htm; Colour selector; http://www.hawkinswatts.com/prod_cols.htm#

Diana, Colour Impact Configurator: http://www.diana-food.com/colourimpact/colourimpact_colour.html

Forms of colourings available: Univar colours, http://www.univarcolour.com/colours_food.php

Aluminium lakes: FAO aluminium lakes of colouring matters, http://www.fao.org/ag/agn/jecfa-additives/specs/monograph3/additive-013.pdf

Coloured coatings: Viskase, https://www.yumpu.com/en/document/view/4369432/viscoat-color-master-tds-website-public-viskase

Pearlescent colours: Candurin, http://www.innovadex.com/documents/1128282.pdf?bs=4370&b=196682&st=1&sl=27207194&crit=a2V5d29yZDpbY29sb3Vyc10%3d&k=colours|color|colors|colour

Clouding agents: *The Soft Drinks Companion*, Maurice Shachman

'There is a difficult legislative boundary between a food colour additive and a colouring food': *Guidelines on approaches to the replacement of Tartrazine, Allura Red, Ponceau 4R, Quinoline Yellow, Sunset Yellow and Carmoisine in food and beverages*, available at: http://www.food.gov.uk/sites/default/files/multimedia/pdfs/publication/guidelinessotonsixcolours.pdf

Definition of 'colouring food': EU guidance on the notes on the classification of food extracts with colouring properties, http://ec.europa.eu/food/food/fAEF/additives/docs/guidance_en.pdf

Blood as a colouring food: http://www.vepro.biz/en/colourant-54.htm

PSE meat: FAO Guidelines for Humane Handling, Transport and Slaughter, Chapter 2, http://www.fao.org/docrep/003/x6909e/x6909e04.htm

Chapter 10

'Transglutaminase, an enzyme ... is now widespread in meat processing': BDF, Leading food solutions brochure, Probind TX

'Transglutaminase ... transforms worthless cuts of meat or fish': *ibid*

Meat glue: Ajinomoto Activa, http://www.amazon.com/Ajinomoto-Activa-Transglutaminase-Meat-2-2-Pound/dp/B003EX2ECM; http://www.amazon.com/Ajinomoto-Activa-Transglutaminase-Meat-2-2-Pound/dp/B003EX2ECM

Salami Dry Express B9: FI Daily 2013, page 46

Transglutaminase EU regulatory position: *ibid*

Soapy taste of phosphates: Nassau Foods, Technical information sheet: Phosphates in meat products, http://www.nassaufoods.com/index.php?content=linksresources

Phosphates: Prayon, Phosphates for meat and poultry products brochure

Phosphate dipping of fish fillets: *ibid*

FSA scallop testing: November 2002, http://food.gov.uk/multimedia/pdfs/30scampi.pdf

Carrageenan: PT Algalindo Perdana brochure

'tightly bind added water in processed meat products': Fiber-Star, *The Citri-Fi Users Guide*

'One company with a buoyant business in the field': InterFiber, Unicell fibers improve your meat products

Swelite®: Cosucra, Texture improvement of restructured frozen poultry products: Swelite® Technical Paper

Ultra Create: National Starch Food Innovation product brochure

'Soya protein is another useful 'meat extender' for manufacturers': FAO technology of production of edible flours and protein products from soya beans, 7-5-1 Meat extenders, http://www.fao.org/docrep/t0532e/t0532e08.htm

Collagen: 'BHJ How do functional proteins work?' http://www.bhj.com/News/Newsarchive/2013/News/How%20proteins%20work.aspx

'Canned, pasteurised and stored at room temperature': http://www.bhj.co.uk/Functional-Proteins/Functional-Protiens-Stock/Info-Material.aspx

'As one supplier of chemicals to food manufacturers': Brenntag, Shared Values – Shared Success: Proteins brochure

FPH and HFP: Application of additives in chilled and frozen white fish fillets, Magnea Gudrun Karlsdottir, September 2009, http://skemman.is/stream/get/1946/4131/11834/1/Master_thesis_final2_Magnea.pdf

'In the words of one company, "beef up their sales": BHJ Scanpro flyer, http://issuu.com/bhjdk/docs/beef_protein_flyer?e=2315981/3478979

'A manufacturer pays £1.85 a kilo': *ibid*

'As one protein company puts it': Proliant Meat Ingredients, Functional proteins, http://www.proliantmeatingredients.com/products.aspx?catid=117&rootid=117&countryid=125

Veos plasma proteins: http://www.vepro.biz/en/plasma-12.htm

Veos globin: http://www.vepro.biz/en/globin-52.htm

'Sold through a worldwide sales network': *Food Ingredients Daily Europe*, 2013, page 17

'A recipe for hot dogs': Interfiber®, Fibers of nature brochure

'A recipe for bacon brine': Dr Harnisch, Better bacon on the table, http://www.harnisch.com/uploads/tx_harnisch/fmt_4_12_14-16.pdf

Tumbling/injecting meat equipment: FAO meat processing technology for small-to medium-scale producers ..., http://www.fao.org/docrep/010/ai407e/ai407e14.htm; http://www.fao.org/docrep/010/ai407e/ai407e04.htm

'Without the hassle of blisters': Sabofa, Flavour jet, http://www.youtube.com/watch?v=eC6qJWe5Ul4

'12,000 chickens an hour': *ibid*

'When the *Guardian* ... calculated': *Guardian*, 7 December 2013, Supermarket customers buying frozen chicken pay 20 per cent for water and additives

Subsequent *Daily Mail* investigation: *Daily Mail*, 9 December 2013, How supermarkets charge you £1.54 a kilo for water added to bulk up chicken

Chapter 11

'Since their development in the 1940s, modified food starches have become a vital part of the food industry': 'Modified Food Starches, Why, What, Where and How', Joseph M. Light, National Starch and Chemical Co., adapted from a presentation at the symposium on Modified Food Starches at AACC's 74th Annual Meeting in Washington, DC, 29 October to 2 November 1989, http://sa.foodinnovation.com/pdfs/modified.pdf

'adhesion, antistaling, binding': *ibid*, http://www.intechopen.com/download/get/type/pdfs/id/34060

'Food manufacturers generally prefer starches': 'Modified Starches and Their Usages', Abbas, Khalil, Hussin, *Journal of Agricultural Science*, Vol. 2, No. 2, June 2010, http://www.ccsenet.org/journal/index.php/jas/article/viewFile/4069/4919

Various techniques for modifying starch, Neelan/Veejay/Lalit in *International Research Journal of Pharmacy*, 2230–8407, 9 March 2012, http://www.irjponline.com/admin/php/uploads/1061_pdf.pdf

'The starch in canned soups [and] ... a factory pizza': What is modified starch? Roy Ballam, British Nutrition Foundation, *Independent*, 11 October 1998, http://www.independent.co.uk/arts-entertainment/food-drink-food-for-thought-what-is-modified-starch-1177698.html

Methods for modifying starch: Physical and/or chemical modifications of starch by thermoplastic extrusion, Clerici, March 2012, http://www.intechopen.com/download/get/type/pdfs/id/34060

'Speciality starches continue to outpace unmodified starches': Speciality starches for snack foods, M.G. Sajilata, Rekha S. Singhal, Department of Food and Fermentation Technology, Institute of Chemical Technology, University of Mumbai, http://www.aseanfood.info/articles/11020956.pdf

'Like you, we're committed to keeping costs low': National Starch, 'Consider the secrets of cost-effective innovation', http://www.foodinnovation.com/valuematters/index.html

'The addition of starch allows opulently labelled 'all butter' biscuits or croissants to contain less butter': Ulrick&Short Ingredients, 'Making the biscuit', http://www.ulrickandshort.com/news%20pdfs/PR57a%20Biscuit%20World.pdf

Delyte: What is Delyte? http://www.ulrickandshort.com/delyte.html

'Once you've created the structure with your base starch': National Starch N-dulge co-texturiser brochure

'Our specialty solutions mimic the organoleptic qualities of fat': National Starch, Starch-based solutions for cost effective convenience, http://www.foodinnovation.com/Downloads/Company/100034VMSavoryR0.pdf

'Starch can stand in for 30% of the cream in a ready-meal spaghetti carbonara': Precisa cream substitutes product brochure

'And make redundant at least 25% of the tomato paste': Tate & Lyle press release, 28 October 2013, http://www.tateandlyle.presscentre.com/Press-releases/Pulp-Performance-Tate-Lyle-Launches-PULPIZ-Pulp-Extender-Delivers-Key-Replacement-Advantages-in-43f.aspx

'It allows manufacturers to reduce the margarine in puff pastry by a fifth': Culinar Volume; Speciality starch for puff pastry margarine brochure; Cindy Haze, *Food Product Design*, 19 October 2009, http://www.foodproductdesign.com/articles/2009/10/ingredient-economics.aspx?pg=5http://www.dairyreporter.com/Ingredients/Emerging-market-processed-cheese-starch-demand-up-Ingredion

'Up to 40% of tomato/vegetable solids in soups and sauces': Introducing Precisa, http://www.foodinnovation.com/Downloads/Company/090061_PRECISA_Cling_flyer.pdf

'Food technologists are a creative, but miserly, crowd': A ratio of up to 10:1, National Starch, Lower cost liquid foods, http://www.foodinnovation.com/valuematters/sauces-soups-dressings-dips.html

'As the spokesman for one dairy company notes': Torben Jensen, Application Manager at Arla Foods Ingredients, http://www.naturalproductsinsider.com/news/2013/01/arla-nutrilac-protein-solution.aspx

Arla Foods Ingredients: Less milk more cheese, http://www.arlafoodsingredients.com/applications/application-overview/cheese/cream-cheese/

Arla Foods Ingredients; Tap into the trend for Greek yogurt http://www.arlafoodsingredients.com/upload/arla%20ingredients/applications/fmp/greek%20yoghurt/arla_greekyog_infographic_v2.pdf

Ingredion: Achieve rich, creamy texture in Greek-style yogurt with a cost effective approach: http://www.foodinnovation.com/foodinnovation/en-us/RegForms/Documents/Ingredion%20Greek%20Yogurt%20White%20Paper-Final.pdf

'"Cereal-based starches such as corn and wheat"': AACC International Starch Handbook, chapter 5, Matching starches to applications http://www.aaccnet.org/publications/plexus/cfwplexus/pub/2012/StarchHandbkCh5.pdf

'"They are used as bland-tasting functional ingredients"': Novozymes brochure; Enzymes at work http://www.novozymes.com/en/about-us/brochures/Documents/Enzymes_at_work.pdf

'"The bland taste of potato starches"': Application improvements, Emsland potato starch brochure

'Rather than avoiding starchy foods, it's better to try and base your meals on them': FSA Scotland, Starchy foods, http://www.eatwellscotland.org/healthydiet/nutritionessentials/starchfoods/index.html

'Starchy foods ... have been hyped by public health agencies': NHS Choice, Starchy foods, http://www.nhs.uk/Livewell/Goodfood/Pages/starchy-foods.aspx

Asda Extra Light Mayonnaise: Ingredient listing taken from Asda website, 7 October 2013

Chapter 12

'Enzymes ... are one of the leading "green chemistry" technologies': Enzyme Technical Association, Environmental/Sustainability, http://www.enzymeassociation.org/?page_id=91

'Enzymes are best known for their industrial applications': Enzyme Technical Association, Enzymes: A Primer on Use and Benefits, Today and Tomorrow, http://www.enzymeassociation.org/wp-content/uploads/2013/09/benefits_paper.pdf

'The Enzyme Technical Association ... explains the "enzyme advantage"': Enzyme Technical Association, Enzymes: A Primer on Uses and Benefits, Today and Tomorrow, http://www.enzymeassociation.org/wp-content/uploads/2013/09/benefits_paper.pdf

'Nearly all commercially prepared foods contain at least one ingredient that has been made with [enzymes]': Enzyme Technical Association, Food, http://www.enzymeassociation.org/?page_id=44

Enzymes as catalysts: Enzyme Technical Association, About enzymes file:///Users/joanna/Desktop/About%20Enzymes%20Enzyme%20Tech%20Assoc.webarchive

'Some of them perform their task up to five million times a minute': EUFIC, 'Food without enzymes?', http://www.eufic.org/article/en/page/RARCHIVE/expid/review-food-without-enzymes/

'Enzymes ... do "the work of a small factory"': Biocatalysts brochure, Our Vision

'By using certain amylases during fermentation': Enzymes in the fruit juice, wine, brewing and distilling industries, Enzyme Technology, http://www1.lsbu.ac.uk/water/enztech/fruitjuice.html

'High fructose corn syrup ... is now produced using enzymes': Enzyme Technical Association, Enzymes: A Primer on Use and Benefits, Today and Tomorrow, http://www.enzymeassociation.org/wp-content/uploads/2013/09/benefits_paper.pdf

'To ensure that bakery goods': *ibid*

'Fruit salads are often processed with pectinase': Health Canada, List of Permitted Food Enzymes, http://www.hc-sc.gc.ca/fn-an/securit/addit/list/5-enzymes-eng.php

'Amyloglucosidase will give industrial bread an evenly brown crust': Enzyme Technical Association, Enzymes: A Primer on Use and Benefits, Today and Tomorrow, http://www.enzymeassociation.org/wp-content/uploads/2013/09/benefits_paper.pdf

'Maltogenic amylase will delay the rate at which it stales': Andrew Whitley, *Bread Matters*, Fourth Estate, 2009, p. 12

'A dash of pectin methylesterase will make your frozen raspberries and green beans firmer': The use of enzymes in improving fruit firmness, Novozymes product brochure

Lipases and cheese flavour: *ibid*

Juice and pectinase: *ibid*

Pectinase: Biocatalysts: The use of enzymes in improving fruit firmness, Company factsheet

'Fresh peeled citrus fruit segments destined for ready-to-eat fruit salads are often processed with pectinase': Novozymes, Enzymes at work 6.7.3, http://www.novozymes.com/en/about-us/brochures/Documents/Enzymes_at_work.pdf

VERON® xTender: AB Enzymes, http://www.abenzymes.com/products/baking/veron-xtender

Maxipro HSP: Fi Europe Excellence Awards 2013, http://www.healthgauge.com/read/fi-europe-excellence-awards-2013/

'DSM says that Maxipro HSP has "excellent gelation and waterbinding properties"': DSM press release, 9 October 2013, http://www.dsm.com/content/dam/dsm/cworld/en_US/documents/2013-10-09-maxipro-at-fie-innovation-in-protein-isolation.pdf

'Subtilisin is another enzyme employed to reinvent red blood cells': Applications of proteases in the food industry, Enzyme Technology, http://www1.lsbu.ac.uk/water/enztech/proteases.html

'One feed enzymes company commentator explains': Alex Ford, Enzymes and their use in animal feed, BioResource International, Inc., http://briworldwide.com/enzymes-and-their-use-in-animal-feed/#sthash.AYD8sGM5.ZLpFOT4G.dpbs

'Chickens fed a two per cent lower protein diet': *ibid*

'Enzymes also improve the profile of cheaper animals feeds, such as 'feather meal': BioResource International, Inc., Valkerase® brochure, http://www.briworldwide.com/wp-content/uploads/2011/10/Valkerase-Brochure.pdf

Produced from coarse and fine scrap-bone residues from the mechanical fleshing of beef, pig, turkey, or chicken bones, Novozymes, Enzymes at work 6.6.2, http://www.novozymes.com/en/about-us/brochures/Documents/Enzymes_at_work.pdf

'"The meat slurry produced," one authority explains, "is used in canned meats and soups"': Applications of proteases in the food industry; Enzymes in the fruit juice, wine, brewing and distilling industries, Enzyme Technology, Available at: http://www1.lsbu.ac.uk/water/enztech/proteases.html

Papain enzyme injected into their jugular vein: *ibid*

'Over 150 enzymes are now in being used in the food and drink industry': European Commission, Collection of information on enzymes 4, http://ec.europa.eu/environment/archives/dansub/pdfs/enzymerepcomplete.pdf

'The importance of enzymes in everyday life is one of today's best-kept secrets': Enzyme Technical Association, Enzymes: A Primer on Use and Benefits, Today and Tomorrow, http://www.enzymeassociation.org/wp-content/uploads/2013/09/benefits_paper.pdf

'"They shall be present in the food in the form of a residue"': Europa summaries, Food enzymes, http://europa.eu/legislation_summaries/consumers/product_labelling_and_packaging/sa0004_en.html

'"The industry will kick and scream"': *Food Manufacture*, 9 August 2012 http://www.foodmanufacture.co.uk/Regulation/EU-enzyme-scrutiny-could-open-up-GM-can-of-worms

'Purified enzymes do not lose their properties': EUFIC, Enzymes make clean green food, http://www.eufic.org/article/en/artid/enymes-clean-green-food/

GM enzymes: European Commission, Collection of information on enzymes 3.3.1.2, http://ec.europa.eu/environment/archives/dansub/pdfs/enzymerepcomplete.pdf

Created by fermenting microorganisms, or extracted and purified from plant or animal sources: Enzyme Technical Association, About enzymes

Sources for lipase: Health Canada, List of permitted food enzymes, http://www.hc-sc.gc.ca/fn-an/securit/addit/list/5-enzymes-eng.php

'Some of the most common GM enzymes in our food': EUFIC, Modern Biotechnology in Food, Applications of food biotechnology: enzymes, http://www.eufic.org/article/en/rid/modern-biotechnology-food-enzymes/

Asparaginase and E. coli: Sources of enzymes; Enzymes in the fruit juice, wine, brewing and distilling industries, Enzyme Technology, Available at http://www1.lsbu.ac.uk/water/enztech/sources.html

'"For the food enzyme industry, all of nature is a chemistry set"': Andrew Whitley, *Bread Matters*, Fourth Estate, 2009, p. 17

Capacities of up to 150,000 litres: EUFIC, Modern Biotechnology in Food, Applications of food biotechnology: enzymes, http://www.eufic.org/article/en/rid/modern-biotechnology-food-enzymes/

'"Details of components used in industrial-scale fermentation broths for enzyme production are not readily obtained"': *ibid*

Likely ingredients include waste materials and by-products from the food and agricultural industries: *ibid*

'"Safety assurance has a short shelf life"': Andrew Whitley, *Bread Matters*, Fourth Estate, 2009, p. 14

'The research team made a point of noting': European Commission, Collection of information on enzymes, 2.2 Terms of reference, http://ec.europa.eu/environment/archives/dansub/pdfs/enzymerepcomplete.pdf

Safety of enzymes: Safety and regulatory aspects of enzyme use, Enzyme Technology: Enzymes in the fruit juice, wine, brewing and distilling industries, *Enzyme Technology*, Available at: http://www1.lsbu.ac.uk/water/enztech/index.html

European Commission, Collection of information on enzymes 11.2.5/6.7.3, http://ec.europa.eu/environment/archives/dansub/pdfs/enzymerepcomplete.pdf

'20 per cent of its allergenicity can survive in the crusts of bread': Sander, I., Raulf-Heimsoth, M., Van Kampen, V., Baur, X (2000) 'Is fungal amylase in bread and allergen?' *Clin Exp*

Allergy, 200 April:30(4):560–5 http://www.ncbi.nlm.nih.gov/pubmed/10718854

'It can generate the part of the epitope [part of molecule] responsible for coeliac disease': Gerrard J., & Sutton K. (2005) 'Addition of transglutaminase to cereal products may generate the epitope responsible for coeliac disease', *Trends Food Sci Technol* 16, 510–512, http://www.researchgate.net/publication/240425204_Addition_of_transglutaminase_to_cereal_products_may_generate_the_epitope_responsible_for_coeliac_disease

'The concept of acceptable risk': EUFIC, Enzymes make clean green food, http://www.eufic.org/article/en/artid/enymes-clean-green-food/

Chapter 13

'Over 80 additives that have a preservative effect are approved in Europe': Using preservatives, FAIA, http://www.understandingfoodadditives.org/pages/ch2p5-3.htm

'Many of them are just "synthetic copies of the natural [preservative] products that are present in nature"': *ibid*

'Such preservatives are ... "quite chemical in nature"': Wayne Morley of Leatherhead Food Research, 'Preservative perceptions; Consumer demand for natural is serious, but challenges remain', *Food Navigator*, 3 December 2013, http://www.foodnavigator.com/Science-Nutrition/Preservative-perceptions-Consumer-demand-for-natural-is-serious-but-challenges-remain

'The additive industry itself admits that sulphites ... can trigger breathing difficulties': Preservatives to keep food longer – and safer, http://www.eufic.org/article/en/food-safety-quality/food-additives/artid/preservatives-food-longer-safer/

'Consumption of the preservative sodium benzoate ... could be linked to increased hyperactivity': Food colours and hyperactivity, https://www.food.gov.uk/science/additives/foodcolours

‘Nitrosamines, which are potent carcinogens’: R. A. Winter, *Consumer’s Dictionary of Food Additives* (7th edn), Random House, 2009, pp. 382–385.

Difference between vitamin C and ascorbic acid: Natural Whole Food Vitamins: Ascorbic Acid Is Not Vitamin C, The *Doctor Within*, http://www.thedoctorwithin.com/vitaminc/ascorbic-acid-is-not-vitamin-c/

‘Ascorbic acid is made industrially ... by the fermentation of GM corn’: Going non-GMO in dietary supplements, ‘The supply community is not there with us yet’, say manufacturers, Nutra ingredients-USA.com, 5 June 2013, http://www.nutraingredients-usa.com/Markets/Going-non-GMO-in-dietary-supplements-The-supply-community-is-not-there-with-us-yet-say-manufacturers

‘Synthetic vitamins are not as well absorbed in the body as natural ones’: ‘The Truth About Vitamins in Nutritional Supplements’, Doctor’s Research, http://www.doctorsresearch.com/articles4.html

‘An ingredient in embalming fluid and jet fuel’: Wikipedia, Butylated hydroxytoluene, http://en.wikipedia.org/wiki/Butylated_hydroxytoluene

‘A common component of rubber and petroleum products’: Wikipedia, Butylated hydroxyanisole, http://en.wikipedia.org/wiki/Butylated_hydroxyanisole

‘Which finds another purpose in the making of varnish’: Wikipedia, tert-Butylhydroquinone, http://en.wikipedia.org/wiki/Tert-Butylhydroquinone

EUFIC functions as a food industry lobby group: http://www.powerbase.info/index.php/European_Food_Information_Council

‘Under the tabloid-style headline “Kitchen sink squalor”’: NHS Choices, Food and hygiene facts, http://www.nhs.uk/Livewell/homehygiene/Pages/food-and-home-hygiene-facts.aspx

'A factory is what we call a hygienic, efficient place': @123db_GEEK retweeted by @retailmentoring, 31 May 2014

'The profitability is directly impacted in a positive direction': PLT Health Solutions, Shelf Life Extension, http://www.plthealth.com/food-beverage/shelf-life-extension

'There are no improvements ... that will ... increase your bottom line as much as shelf life extension': Gillco Ingredients, Extend Shelf Life, http://www.gillco.com/idea_shelf-life.php

Small firms pressured to use longer shelf-life dates, *Food Manufacture*, 24 July 2013, http://www.foodmanufacture.co.uk/Food-Safety/Small-meat-firms-pressured-to-use-longer-shelf-life-dates

'Often in tandem with modified atmosphere packaging': http://www.modifiedatmospherepackaging.com

'Now foods packaged using MAP must be labelled': Chilled Food Association, Modified Atmosphere Packaging and vitamin levels in salads, http://www.chilledfood.org/MEDIA/POSITION+STATEMENTS/modified-atmosphere-packaging-map-and-vitamin-levels-in-salads-

MAP and pre-baked pitta breads: Modified Atmosphere Packaging of Bread Products, http://modifiedatmospherepackaging.com/Applications/Modified-atmosphere-packaging-bread-products

'Some bakery goods can be given a shelf life of up to 6 months': *ibid*

'MAP can add 5 or 6 days to the shelf life of a sandwich': Modified Atmosphere Packaging of Prepared Foods and Ready Meals, http://modifiedatmospherepackaging.com/Applications/Modified-atmosphere-packaging-ready-meals

Use-by date extension of ready meal using MAP: *ibid*

Oxidative warmed-over flavour: *ibid*

WOF: Warmed-over flavor a processing challenge, http://www.highbeam.com/doc/1G1-10007439I.html

MAP and 'case ready' meat: Modified Atmosphere Packaging of Fresh Meat; http://www.modifiedatmospherepackaging.com/Applications/Modified-atmosphere-packaging-fresh-meat.aspx

Lamb sent frozen from New Zealand: ITN *Tonight*, July 2014

Dansensor: Quality Control and Quality Assurance of Modified Atmosphere Packaging – gain extended food shelf life, http://modifiedatmospherepackaging.com/QC-QA-of-Modified-Atmosphere-Packaging-for-extended-food-shelf-life

What scientists refer to as 'wounded' tissues: Porta, R. *et al.*, Edible Coating as Packaging Strategy to Extend the Shelf-life of Fresh-Cut Fruits and Vegetables, J Biotechnol Biomater (2013); 3:e124. doi: 10.4172/2155-952X.1000e124, http://omicsonline.org/open-access/edible-coating-as-packaging-strategy-to-extend-the-shelflife-of-freshcut-fruits-and-vegetables-2155-952X-3-e124.php?aid=22423#5

'Prepared vegetable suppliers can add up to 8 days to the use-by date of salad leaves': Modified Atmosphere Packaging for Fresh Fruits and Vegetables, http://modifiedatmospherepackaging.com/Applications/Modified-atmosphere-packaging-fruit-vegetables

'A Jacuzzi-style wash tank': Agricoat, NatureSeal FS product brochure

'Fruit acids ... are often also included in the mix': Chilled Food Association, Produce washing, http://www.chilledfood.org/MEDIA/POSITION+STATEMENTS/produce-washing-

NatureSeal FS: Agricoat, NatureSeal FS product brochure

Edible films and coatings: Valencia-Chamorro, S. A., *et al.*, 'Antimicrobial edible films and coatings for fresh and minimally processed fruits and vegetables': a review, *Crit Rev Food Sci Nutr* (2011); 51: 872–900, http://www.ncbi.nlm.nih.gov/pubmed/21888536

eatFresh-FC and Grow Green Industries: 'The Safe, Healthy Solution For Kitchens, Schools And More', http://eatcleaner.com/commercial

Edible coating technologies for pre- and post-harvest protection: Agricoat, NatureSeal FS product brochure

Semperfresh: *ibid*

'Known in the food preservation business as "smart" or "intelligent' films": FDA, Food, Chapter VI. Microbiological Safety of Controlled and Modified Atmosphere Packaging of Fresh and Fresh-Cut Produce, Section 1.3 Films used in MAP, http://www.fda.gov/Food/FoodScienceResearch/SafePracticesforFoodProcesses/ucm091368.htm

'"Can provide a food with a safe product lifetime of as long as two weeks"': No need to get browned off – edible films keep fruit fresh, David Tribe; *The Conversation*, 2 September 2013, http://theconversation.com/no-need-to-get-browned-off-edible-films-keep-fruit-fresh-18150

'A new edible and cook-able meat coating': MeatCoat, http://www.uecbv.eu/doc/MEATCOAT%20article%20-04.06.2013.pdf

MeatCoat cost: Edible 'meat coat' promises to extend shelf life by three days, *The Grocer*, 8 June 2014, http://www.thegrocer.co.uk/fmcg/fresh/edible-meat-coat-promises-to-extend-shelf-life/358202.article

'Carriers for a wide range of artificial additives': Maftoonazad N. I. and Badii F., 'Use of edible films and coatings to extend the shelf life of food products', *Recent Pat Food Nutr Agric* (2009); 1: 162–170, http://www.ncbi.nlm.nih.gov/pubmed/20653537

'A WOF in a 9-day-old treated pork patty is reduced': 'Fighting Warmed-Over Flavor'; *Food Product Design*: Foodservice Focus – November 2000, http://www.foodproductdesign.com/articles/2000/11/food-product-design-foodservice-focus-november.aspx

XFresh: Zeelandia: Prolong shelf life and improve freshness with these enzyme-based fresheners for cakes, http://www.zeelandia.com/innovation/end-product-performance/freshness-and-shelf-life/xfresh

Verdad F41: Corbion Purac product brochure, http://www.purac.com/EN/Food/Markets/Meat_poultry_and_fish/Clean-label-solutions/Verdad-F.aspx

NaturFORT and Fortium: Kemin product brochure

BioVia™ YM 10: Danisco, The power of 'natural', http://cdn.danisco.com/fileadmin/user_upload/danisco/documents/biovia-brochure.pdf

Ecoprol 2002: Somerex product brochure

'"A disaster waiting to happen"': Marty Mitchell of the Refrigerated Foods Association, 'Chilled foods minus synthetic preservatives: A "natural" disaster waiting to happen?' *Food Navigator*, 28 April 2011, http://www.foodnavigator-usa.com/R-D/Chilled-foods-minus-synthetic-preservatives-A-natural-disaster-waiting-to-happen

'The food scientist Dr Robert L. Shewfelt coined the term "fresh-like"': Shewfelt R. L., 'Quality of minimally processed fruits and vegetables', *J Food Qual* (1987); 10: 143–156

Chapter 14

Tweet to Asda: @Dastardly_Pants, 26 April 2014, pic.twitter.com/Bh1zcZk6Tc

Bubble pads: Sirane, Dri-Fresh® Soft-Hold™ absorbent cushion pads for fruit, http://www.sirane.com/food-packaging-products/dri-fresh/dri-fresh®-soft-hold™-absorbent-cushion-pads-for-soft-fruit.html

'They provide an 'anti-fog' effect': 21 CFR 178.3130 – 'Antistatic and/or anti-fogging agents in food-packaging materials', Legal Information Unit, Cornell University Law School, http://www.law.cornell.edu/cfr/text/21/178.3130

LiquiGlide: 'LiquiGlide gives foods the slip to reduce waste', *Packaging Digest*, 25 February 2013, http://www.packagingdigest.com/food-packaging/liquiglide-gives-foods-slip-reduce-waste

'Mayonnaise dispensers treated with [LiquGlide]': 'LiquiGlide's coatings to hit shelves in 2015', *Food Production Daily*, 27 February 2014, http://www.foodproductiondaily.com/Packaging/LiquiGlide-s-coatings-to-hit-shelves-in-2015

'Composed of no fewer than seven microscopically thin plastic layers': 'New high oxygen and water barrier multilayer film patented', *Food Packaging*, 29 May 2014, http://www.packagingdigest.com/food-packaging/new-high-oxygen-and-water-barrier-multilayer-film-patented140529; http://www.freshpatents.com/-dt20140515ptan20140134446.php

Concerns over non-stick: 'Nervous about non-stick?' *Good Housekeeping*, http://www.goodhousekeeping.com/product-reviews/cooking-tools/cookware-reviews/nonstick-cookware-safety-facts

Chopping board debate: Plastic and wooden cutting boards, Dean O. Cliver, http://faculty.vetmed.ucdavis.edu/faculty/docliver/Research/cuttingboard.htm

'Over 6,000 chemicals are used to make food packaging': Introduction, Chemical Risk Assessment, *Food Packaging Forum*, 26 February 2014, http://www.foodpackagingforum.org/food-packaging-health/chemical-risk-assessment

Food Packaging Forum: FPF About Us, http://www.foodpackagingforum.org/about-us

'Recently warned that 175 dangerous chemicals are found in food packaging': 'Warning over 175 dangerous chemicals found in food packaging: Substances are linked to cancer, fertility and birth defects', *Daily Mail*, 8 July 2014, http://www.dailymail.co.uk/health/article-2684256/Dangerous-chemicals-food-packaging-linked-cancer-fertility-birth-defects-study-finds.html#ixzz37AaSoVpP

'Food contact substances and chemicals of concern: a comparison of inventories': *Food Additives & Contaminants*: Part A, Volume 31, Issue 8, 2014, http://www.tandfonline.com/doi/full/10.1080/19440049.2014.931600

Chemicals of Concerns (COCs): *ibid*

What the EPA's 'Chemicals of Concern' Plans Really Mean, *Scientific American*, 11 January 2010, http://www.scientificamerican.com/article/epa-chemicals-of-concern-plans

'Food contact materials have long been in the frame as a possible major source of chronic exposure to chemicals': Borcher A. *et al.*, *Food Safety*, *Clin Rev Allergy Immunol* (2010); 39: 95–141, http://www.ncbi.nlm.nih.gov/pubmed/19911313

'Their toxicity can be increased in the presence of other chemicals': Kortenkamp A. *et al.*, 'Low-Level Exposure to Multiple Chemicals: Reason for Human Health Concerns?' *Envir Health Perspect* (2007); 115: 106–114, http://discovery.ucl.ac.uk/1363921/1/KORTENKAMP.LOW.pdf

REACH: The Registration Process, http://www.hse.gov.uk/reach/regprocess.htm

'The dose makes the poison': 'Toxicology: The learning curve', Dan Fagin, *Nature*, 24 October 2012, http://www.nature.com/news/toxicology-the-learning-curve-1.11644

'Bisphenol A possible effects': vom Saal F. S. *et al.*, Chapel Hill bisphenol A expert panel consensus statement, *Reprod Toxicol* (2007); 24: 131–138, http://www.ncbi.nlm.nih.gov/pmc/articles/PMC2967230/

Restrictions on bisphenol A in various countries: *Food Packaging Forum*, Bisphenol A, http://www.foodpackagingforum.org/food-packaging-health/bisphenol-a

Bisphenol A in cancer charity avoidance advice: Tips for Avoiding BPA in Canned Food, Breast Cancer Fund, http://www.breastcancerfund.org/reduce-your-risk/tips/avoid-bpa.html

'Breast Cancer UK has called for a ban on bisphenol A': 'BPA should be banned immediately', says Breast Cancer UK, *Food and Drink Europe*, 24 October 2013, http://www.foodanddrinkeurope.com/Products-Marketing/BPA-should-be-banned-immediately-says-Breast-Cancer-UK/?utm_source=newsletter_weekly&utm_medium=email&utm_campaign=Newsletter%2BWeekly&c=lQa1YdAlYo4Fq84iU4nhQ1z1lFk5tlR2

'The highest levels of certain phthalates have been found in bread': *Food Packaging Forum*, Phthalates, 4 October 2012, http://www.foodpackagingforum.org/food-packaging-health/phthalates

'Tests on animals link these chemicals [phthalates] to reduced fertility, and reproductive and testicular toxicity': *ibid*

'31 per cent of foods tested contained phthalates above the level set in European law': Determination of phthalates in foods and establishing methodology to distinguish their source, FSA, http://www.food.gov.uk/science/research/chemical-safety-research/env-cont/c01048#toc-3

'When scientists ... examined cooked food': Cirillo T, *et al.*, 'Children's Exposure to Di(2-ethylhexyl)phthalate and Dibutylphthalate Plasticizers from School Meals', *J Agric Food Chem* (2011); 59: 10532–10538, http://pubs.acs.org/doi/abs/10.1021/jf2020446

'Nanoparticles ... are increasingly used in food and drink packaging': Alfadul S. M. and Elneshwy A. A., 'Use of nanotechnology in food processing, packaging and safety review', *Afr J Food Agric*, Nutr Dev (2010); 10: 6, 2719–2739

Nanosilver and nanoclays: Nanotechnology for the Food Industry, *Nano Magazine*, http://www.nanomagazine.co.uk/index.php?option=com_content&view=article&id=56%3Ananotechnology-for-the-food-industry&Itemid=151

'Aluminium and silicon nanoparticles migrated from plastic bottles into an acidic medium': Farhoodi M *et al.*, 'Migration of Aluminum and Silicon from PET/Clay Nanocomposite Bottles into Acidic Food Simulant', *Packaging Technology and Science* (2014); 27: 161–168, http://www.safenano.org/KnowledgeBase/CurrentAwareness/ArticleView/tabid/168/ArticleId/433/Researchers-study-potential-migration-of-nanoparticles-from-food-packaging.aspx

'They are about one ten-thousandth the width of a human hair': Institute of Food Science and Technology, Information Statement on Nanotechnology, http://www.ifst.org/nanotechnology

'Nanoscale zinc oxide ... has been found to cause lesions': Scientific Committee on Consumer Safety, Opinion on Zinc oxide (nano form), 2012, http://ec.europa.eu/health/scientific_committees/consumer_safety/docs/sccs_o_103.pdf

'Nanoparticles of titanium dioxide can damage DNA, disrupt cell function, and interfere with the defence activities of the immune system': *Tiny Ingredients, Big Risks:* FOE report on nanotechnology, May 2014, http://libcloud.s3.amazonaws.com/93/25/c/4723/2014_Tiny_Ingredients_Big_Risks_Web.pdf

'Nanoparticles absorbed in the gut may be a factor in the growing prevalence of inflammatory conditions': Microparticles and Crohn's Disease, http://www.nutrition411.com/professional-learning/professional-refreshers/item/29665-microparticles-and-crohns-disease/; http://www.ncbi.nlm.nih.gov/pubmed/17202580

'The European Commission acknowledges that nanoparticles could cause health damage': 4. What are the potential health effects of nanomaterials? Nanomaterials, Level 2, http://ec.europa.eu/health/scientific_committees/opinions_layman/nanomaterials/en/l-2/4.htm

'"Full evaluation of the potential hazards is still to come"': 6. How well can we assess the risks from nanomaterials? Nanomaterials, Level 2, http://ec.europa.eu/health/scientific_committees/opinions_layman/nanomaterials/en/index.htm#6

'National Academy of Sciences warns that "critical gaps" in understanding [of nanoparticles] have been identified': 'With Prevalence of Nanomaterials Rising, Panel Urges Review of Risks', *New York Times*, 25 January 2012, http://www.nytimes.com/2012/01/26/science/nanomaterials-effects-on-health-and-environment-unclear-panel-says.html

'About 400–500 nanopackaging products are estimated to be in use now': 'Future nanopackaging market worth billions, says study', *Food Packaging*, 15 May 2007, http://www.foodproductiondaily.com/Packaging/Future-nanopackaging-market-worth-billions-says-study

'Nanosized titanium dioxide ... in products such as coffee creamer, cookies, cream cheese ...': *Tiny Ingredients, Big Risks:*

FOE report on nanotechnology, May 2014, http://libcloud.s3.amazonaws.com/93/25/c/4723/2014_Tiny_Ingredients_Big_Risks_Web.pdf

'A European Union regulation that requires foods (not packaging) containing nanoparticles to be labelled': Towards reference materials for nanoparticles in food, EU Joint Research Centre, 25 June 2014, https://ec.europa.eu/jrc/en/news/towards-reference-materials-nanoparticles-food

Index

Acknowledgements

I am indebted to a number of people who have given me critical help in getting this book written. Whether that was by guiding me to information, giving me the germ of an idea, reading chapters, sharing their expertise and knowledge, or just by supplying moral support, I am deeply grateful.

Some of these people I am able to credit here: David Azoulay, Lynda Brown, Falko Burkert, Gerry Danby, Sue Lawrence, Robert Linton, Mark Nixon, Donald Reid, Garry Scott, Jim Thomas, Denise Walton, Andrew Whitley. Others I cannot name, lest this might have repercussions for their professional lives.

As always, I count myself as one of the luckiest writers in the world to have Louise Haines as my editor. I so appreciate her calm tenacity, her sound judgement, and her openness to ideas. And neither could I wish for a finer agent than Karolina Sutton, whose instincts and reactions I trust absolutely.